# FOOT NOTES

# FOOT NOTES

## by Michelle Arnot

### Drawings by Jack Crane

Foreword by Suzanne M. Levine, D.P.M.

A DOLPHIN BOOK

Doubleday & Company, Inc.
Garden City, New York

1980

Library of Congress Cataloging in Publication Data

Library of Congress Catalog Card Number 79-7857
ISBN: 0-385-14944-1
Copyright © 1980 by MICHELLE ARNOT
All Rights Reserved
Printed in the United States of America
*First Edition*

*To all people*
*devoted to the improvement of foot care.*

# Foreword

The human foot is an architectural wonder—a delicate formation of 26 bones, none more than 13 inches long.

It is an awesome phenomenon that a person weighing more than 300 pounds and over 7 feet tall can be supported in a fully upright position by his feet and transported by them from one place to another at varying speeds. And it is of profound significance that healthy feet have an over-all salutary effect on our physical and mental well-being. Conversely, as the author states, it is the conviction of both foot specialists and foot sufferers that "when our feet hurt, we hurt all over."

It is estimated that the average adult travels over 1,000 miles a year on his feet. To accomplish this movement without faltering, his ankles and subtalar joints must function properly. Any impairment to the muscles controlling these joints can result in rhythmic gait abnormalities.

Furthermore, because of the intricate angular relationship of the ankle, knee, and hip joints, biomechanical foot defects can cause knee, leg, and calf pain, severe backache, awkward knee instability and "hip-hiking," and even a general disruption to our entire center of gravity.

Beyond the gift of locomotion and the prevention of pain and ungainliness are the immeasurable pleasures that healthy feet enable us to enjoy—the sheer ecstasy of the toddler exploring his new world, the exhilaration of the skier gliding down a slope, the zest of the tennis player maneuvering around the court, the stimulation felt by the golfer, the jogger, or the dancer engaged on foot in their activities. And to fill our more pragmatic needs, we owe yet another debt of gratitude to healthy feet. They allow the police-man to "walk the beat," the hurrying commuter to catch his train, the homemaker to move about the house, and all of us to get out of bed in the morning to start another day.

Unfortunately, not everyone is blessed with healthy feet. A re-cent study by the American Podiatry Association prepared for the United States Department of Health, Education, and Welfare re-vealed that over 10 million Americans suffer from soft-tissue anomalies such as corns, calluses, bunions, and nail disorders or static deformities such as clubfeet, flatfeet, and other malforma-tions. It's estimated that 20 million patients are treated in the United States annually for foot injuries, infections, nondeforming bone conditions, and a host of other foot disorders.

It defies comprehension that, despite these distressing statistics, so little attention is focused on proper foot care, especially in a health-conscious society so amenable to publicizing and practicing the prevention of other health hazards. As a result, certain de-structive fallacies continue to be perpetuated.

One common, erroneous theory, for example, is that new shoes are "supposed" to hurt until they are "broken in." Thus, while the wearer is enduring agonizing discomfort, he is simultaneously abusing his feet.

It is certainly a paradox that many a person preoccupied with the dangers of cigarette smoking, hair sprays, and artificial sweet-eners will ignore the serious health damage that can be caused by ill-fitting shoes or those not suitably constructed for specific activi-ties. Frequently, a person who will abstain from eating favorite foods to control his cholesterol intake will carelessly or unwit-tingly mar his health by selecting a shoe too narrow to accommo-date his foot or one with a heel too high to afford proper balance for walking.

Of course, not all self-induced foot disorders are attributable to the unwise choice of shoes. Many are caused by the individual's unawareness of the amount of stress his feet can withstand. He may therefore fail to condition his feet to tolerate the strenuous demands, for example, of jogging or walking long distances on abrasive concrete or gravel. Other self-inflicted foot disorders may result from an overextended range of motion. Skiers and ballet dancers often sustain injuries from such excessive exertion.

Lamentably, knowledge of things detrimental to foot health usually becomes available to the patient already afflicted and in need of treatment, rather than to the voluntary patient who might avoid affliction through preventive care, for despite the voluminous professional literature pertaining to foot health, there is a conspicuous dearth of information addressed to the lay public.

In *Foot Notes,* Michelle Arnot not only distinguishes herself as an engrossing raconteur and foot historian but also renders the invaluable service of offering useful guidance on the prevention and cure of many persisting foot problems. While not intended as a substitute for professional care, the book is an excellent foot-care reference. The author's erudite yet lively discourse probably won't restore the foot to its unique status as the ultimate sex symbol of eleventh-century China, but it will surely motivate the reader to treat his feet with the care they so well deserve—not only for their intrinsic worth but also for their enhancement of general health and well-being.

SUZANNE M. LEVINE
D.P.M.

# Acknowledgments

The author extends special thanks to the many authorities who made this book possible. Most particularly, she would like to express heartfelt gratitude to the following: Dr. Suzanne Levine and her associate Dr. Robert Kirell for long hours of instruction and encouragement; Miss Mary Brown for her invaluable service as both mentor and shoe authority; Dr. Sidney Zerinsky for all his help on the less orthodox treatments of feet; Dr. William Hamilton and Dr. Murray Weisenfeld for their priceless information on dancing feet; Dr. Richard Schuster for insights on running feet; Dr. Bernard Rosenstein for spending many hours discussing the irregularities of feet and the treatment of arthritis; Dr. Elizabeth Roberts for explaining how the foot works and behaves—or misbehaves; Dr. Malcolm Jacobson and Mr. Jack Hawkins for their expertise on shoes; Dr. Jonathan Zizmor for incisive information on the care of skin disorders; and Dr. Louis Galli and Dr. Josef Geldwert for extensive help on sports medicine. Special thanks are also tendered to the Center for Medical Consumers and Health Care Information which afforded the author many hours of pleasant research and excellent facilities. Finally, the author thanks Janell Walden whose idea resulted in this book.

# Contents

# INTRODUCTION
## Standing Tall

Everything stands on feet: tables, chairs, pianos, and some cameras, to name a few items. In fact, the entire notion of verticality implies the existence of feet. Metaphorically, "both feet on the ground" conveys an upright attitude that is undermined once you're swept off your feet and carried away. "He hadn't a foot to stand on," writes Cicero dismissingly.

Thanks to our feet we have a boundless capacity for mobility. Jogging, roller skating, skiing, tennis—what place would these activities have in the scheme of things without our pedal extremities? Muhammad Ali's high stepping, Rudolf Nureyev's bounds, Olga Korbut's acrobatics also would have been lost without early man's desire to stand upright. No John Travolta swagger or Marilyn Monroe wiggle would have crossed the screen; no Charlie Chaplin waddle would have endeared itself to millions of viewers.

Although walking is no longer extolled as a human privilege, it figures prominently in the intellectual sphere. Pacing to and fro is not just an exercise reserved for expectant fathers; the rhythmic movement seems to set our minds in motion until rugs underfoot are worn thin with thought patterns. Henry David Thoreau, a noted hiker, rhapsodizes, "Every walk is a sort of crusade

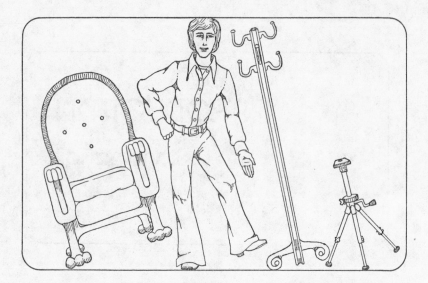

preached by some Peter the Hermit in us to go forth and recon-
quer this Holy Land from the hands of the Infidels." Many sages
derived profound inspiration during their pilgrimages. William
Wordsworth limited his hikes in England's Lake Country to 14
miles a day, whereas Percy Bysshe Shelley gallantly and frequently made the trek from Oxford to London in his student days
—well over 50 miles. Immanuel Kant considered walking one hour
a day sufficient to stimulate his creative philosophic juices; Abraham Lincoln as a young man climbed the Illinois hills in
Springfield on a daily basis.

These days most of our walking is limited to city blocks, and
when we spend a lot of time on our feet, it's usually while standing
in line. Shifting one's weight from left to right foot just isn't the
same uplifting experience as climbing a mountain. In fact, many
of us are forgetting the health benefits derived from using our feet.
Since Roman times, walking has been considered a reliable way to
keep fit. "Before supper, walk a little; after supper, do the same,"
advises Erasmus in the sixteenth century. Thomas Jefferson
echoes this concept: "Walking is the best possible exercise."
Harry Truman appears to have concurred since he made a point
of taking a morning constitutional everyday. The American Heart

Association agrees that "walking briskly—not just strolling—is the simplest and one of the best forms of exercise."

Instead of regarding our feet as the original mode of transportation—holding them up in admiration, marveling at their uncomplaining service—we tend to look down on them as inanimate objects without needs and desires. This current attitude harks back partly to a time when people viewed their feet as a handy measuring tool in the marketplace. It paid to have big feet when buying by the yard—3 feet—since they were used as a rudimentary ruler. And since foot lengths could range up to more than 20 inches, you might find yourself a real bargain. The yard measure was eventually standardized at 36 inches, allegedly the length of King Henry I of England's arm. But the 12-inch foot has been used to measure all manner of entities, for example a foot-candle represents the unit of illumination reaching 12 inches in every direction from one source and the foot-pound is the unit of energy required to lift a 1-pound weight 12 inches.

And yet despite their constant service, we continue to mistreat our feet. Veteran podiatrist Dr. Elizabeth Roberts points out "If you had a blemish on your face, you would have it taken care of promptly. But since your feet don't show, you tend to overlook any problem." Although 98 per cent of us in the United States are born with healthy feet, 80 out of 100 adults will develop foot complaints, mostly self-induced. Dr. Richard Schuster, of the New York College of Podiatric Medicine and a sports medicine pioneer, blames our habit of paving the surfaces we walk on as a major reason. We invest over $200 million each year in over-the-counter foot medications that may or may not work. An estimated 95 per cent of the 500 known foot ailments are traced to ill-designed shoes and improper foot care. Sooner or later, however, we've got to pamper our obedient "dogs" if we want to keep in step.

Apart from transporting mankind, feet have proven quite versatile as a source of inspiration. Dancers and athletes are always aspiring to new heights, while sculptors and painters have painstakingly reproduced the delicate arch, the curled toe. In fact, controversy has traditionally shadowed the foot in the arts. In ancient times, virgin goddesses were depicted with covered feet to protect their chastity. Through the nineteenth century, women's feet were glossed over in painting and literature to maintain propriety. Removing one's shoes was viewed as a seductive gesture inappropriate in a public display.

The Spanish were particularly prudish in this respect—The Roman Catholic hierarchy threatening offenders with excommunication for baring feet. In 1649 Francisco Pacheco wrote: "What could be more foreign from the respect we owe to the purity of Our Lady the Virgin than to paint her sitting down with one of her knees placed over the other, and often with her sacred feet uncovered and naked." Revealing the foot was considered equivalent to a blatant proposition. Francisco Goya was even persuaded to disguise the foot of the Duchess of Alba in one of his portraits of that lady. Her toe had been pointed toward his signature—a suggestive gesture, in the opinion of the censors of the day.

Symbolically the foot dances to many tunes. Pedestal, vehicle, sex symbol—all are contained in that relatively small appendage we stuff thoughtlessly into a shoe. The foot as metaphor emerges even in the Bible. Biblical references often speak of "covering the feet," a vague phrase implying general modesty. Over the centuries the foot evolved into the symbolic image frequently mentioned in parables and proverbs: "All feet tread not in one shoe," "Never tell thy foe that thy feet acheth," "Where your will is ready, your feet are light," "The cat would eat fish and would not wet her feet," "The shoe is now on the other foot." The foot also tickled William Shakespeare's fancy and he included several remarks about feet in his works, among his many references to them being "Men were deceivers ever; / One foot in sea and one on shore, / To one thing constant never." His French contemporary Montaigne says: "To each foot its shoe."

To take a big step in time, eighteenth-century Westerners regarded the foot with great titillation. Any revelation of that appendage was enough to compromise a young lady's reputation. Dresses dragged in the mud rather than show a sexy little foot. Ladies of the nineteenth century displayed more daring—and men described what they saw. "Feet like sunny gems on an English green," writes Lord Tennyson; Algernon Charles Swinburne exhibits equal fervor: "Bind on thy sandals . . . / Over the splen-

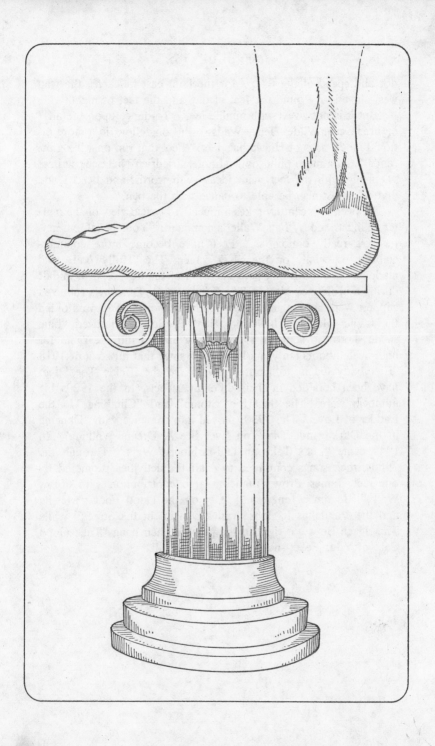

dor and speed of thy feet; / for the faint east quickens, the wan
west shivers, / Round the feet of day and the feet of night."

"But it is not sweet with nimble feet / To dance upon the air!"
mourns Oscar Wilde. Henry Wadsworth Longfellow, in a more ra-
tional mode, says of Hiawatha's feet: "Feet that run on willing er-
rands!" On a more philosophical note, Friedrich Nietzsche writes:
"Dancing with the feet, with ideas, with words, and need I add
that one must also be able to dance with the pen?"

The twentieth century takes a much less lyrical view of the matter as illustrated by Fats Waller's comment: "Your pedal extremities are really obnoxious." Feet have become more commer-
cialized, especially on the silver screen. The "Hollywood foot"
made its debut with that pert extension of the leg posed in midair
during a prolonged kiss. In *The Wizard of Oz* Dorothy's ruby red
slippers were her magic ticket to Kansas. *The Red Shoes* unfolded
the tragic tale of a ballerina. Elvis Presley popularized "blue
suede shoes" in song in 1956; Nancy Sinatra did the same for
high-heeled boots ten years later. Ever since that hit song of 1918
"Ev'rybody Ought to Know How to Do the Tickle Toe," feet
have been heralded in their different aspects. In the 1920s big
numbers were "The Sugarfoot Stomp" and "Climbing Up the
Ladder of Love." The 1930s moved into romance with "Dancing
in the Dark" and "Did You Ever See A Dream Walking?" In
1949 came "Let's Take an Old-fashioned Walk." Through the
1960s, rock songs continued to exalt the activities promoted by
our feet. James Brown made a large contribution with "Slow
Walk," "Joggin' Along," and "Get on the Good Foot"; Martha
and the Vandellas let loose with "Dancin' in the Street," while
The Beach Boys got right to the point in their song "Take Good
Care of Your Feet"—not a bad dictum at all.

# FOOT NOTES

# WHAT'S IN A FOOT?

*"The important feature about earliest man was not so much his brains, but his feet."*
WESTON LA BARRE, ANTHROPOLOGIST, DUKE UNIVERSITY

Consider how much distance you travel on your feet: during the average seventy-year life-span some 70,000 miles are covered—which translates into 2.5 times around the world. The average adult walks well over 1,000 miles a year and yet we hesitate to give our feet the credit they so sorely deserve.

When Leonardo da Vinci called the foot "a masterpiece of engineering and a work of art," he was hardly exaggerating. That size-8 or -10 foot contains *26* small bones plus 2 sesamoids (even smaller bones), *114* ligaments, and *20* muscles. Durable connective layers of tissue, many yards of blood vessels, and an intricate network of nerves join the components of the foot together; the product is finally packaged in layers of skin and then studded with toenails.

The foot houses about the same number of bones as the hand (26 and 27 respectively); together the hands and feet contain half the bones in the body. In fanlike formation, the bones extend in

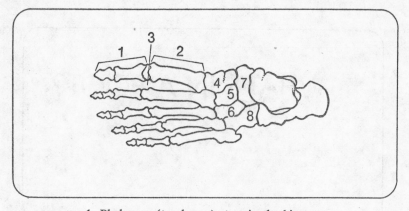

1. Phalanges (toe bones); two in the big toe,
three in each other toe.　2. Metatarsal bones.
3. Web space.　4,5,6. Cuneiform bones.
7. Navicular bone.　8. Cuboid bone.

five rays from the fifth, or little, toe to the hallux, or big toe. There are three phalanges (toe bones) in each toe except the big one, which contains only two. The five metatarsals, the long bones that extend the length of the foot, are connected by ligaments to the toes. "Web space" between the metatarsals creates a passageway for nerves and vessels to pass into the toes. The three cuneiform (wedge-shaped) bones build the midfoot, which helps to stabilize and support body weight. In a way, the midfoot is a bridge with the ligaments serving as cables, and just as in the case of a bridge, we depend on the integrity of its structure for transportation. With the navicular (boat-shaped) and cuboid bones, the cuneiforms help to build the longitudinal arch which reaches from heel to ball. We also know this arch as the "instep"—the layman's term; it is simply the underside, or plantar, aspect of the midfoot. "Plantar" refers to the sole of the foot.

Depending upon genetic factors, your longitudinal arch may be high or low. Supported and supplied with go-ahead power by the muscles, a strong "spring" ligament that prevents shocks to the spine, and the plantar fascia, a band of connective tissue works as a lever. The two arches in the foot—one lengthwise and one across —provide the elastic spring that gives bounce to our steps. The

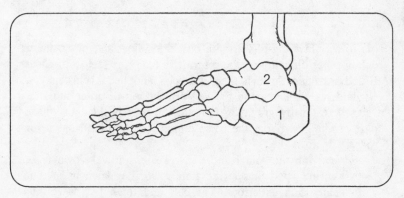

1. Calcaneus (heel). 2. Talus (ankle).

metatarsal arch that spans the ball of the foot stretches the term "arch"; actually, any visible curve here flattens out somewhat during weight bearing in the healthy foot.

The heel, or calcaneus, is the largest bone in the foot and often bears the brunt of our weight. For this reason, protective layers of fat, here as well as on the outside border and ball of the foot, cushion the impact of each footstep. Up-and-down leverage is supplied by the ankle, or talus, while the in-and-out motion originates in the subtalar joint directly below. The subtalar joint also endows us with the ability to tread uneven turf. The joints in the foot account for the range of motions and are located between articulating bones. The muscles in turn control these motions. With the cooperation of tendons, muscles are responsible for the dynamic support of the foot; bones, ligaments, and tissue provide the static elements. Extrinsic muscles in the leg provide strength and motion from above. They connect to the heel via the Achilles tendon, a term dating back to the ancient Greek mythic hero with the vulnerable heel. Intrinsic muscles are found in the foot itself. The only prominent muscle—musculus extensor digitorum brevis—appears in front of the ankle and is often mistaken for an edema (abnormal swelling). Never fear: as long as it remains the same size, rest assured that if it is large, it is simply the sign of a strong foot.

Normal activity of the muscles assists the blood circulation in the feet by "massaging" the blood vessels. Gravity, that unbeata-

ble force, plays tug-of-war with our blood flow and often the circulation has difficulty on the return trip from the feet to the heart.
Blood traveling through the superficial and deep veins may get
waylaid; varicose veins in the legs are the out-of-order superficial
veins defeated by gravity. After all, the foot is the most distant
part of our body from the heart pump and the blood has a long
round trip to make.

Nerves from the spinal and pelvic regions travel down to our
feet to ensure good muscle function. Also they keep us in touch
with whatever is underfoot. The calf and thigh nerves continue
into the feet as the main nerves. Their patterns allow the doctors
to inject anesthetics above the foot, in parts of the ankle, in order
to numb the sole.

All these foot components are wrapped in thick and thin layers
of skin. The thin variety is simply an extension of our normal
body wrap and contains hair follicles and oil glands. Thick skin
tends to develop into callus, sometimes five layers deep on the
sole, in protective formation. Ridges on this heavy surface provide
the traction we need to move forward.

With caloric energy as fuel, the major function of this amazing
foot is to provide locomotion. In the walking process it alternates
between two complementary phases: locking and unlocking. Each
step means losing and regaining balance as we shift from the
stance phase on the ground to the swing phase when the foot is in
midair. Basically, the foot moves as a flexible entity in a skin bag
that conforms to variable surfaces. As the foot comes down upon
a surface, it acts as a shock absorber. In the second phase, it becomes a rigid structure supporting body weight in motion. At no
point is the total foot flat on the ground during gait. Any variation
in this complex system means faulty foot function. If excess energy overloads the vulnerable foot, we risk damaging those fragile
toe bones. Or if shock absorption is diminished by faulty ligaments, pain may radiate all the way up to our spine.

While we would hope to exert ideal pressure on our feet during
each phase, we have to take into consideration the variety of walking patterns. Most people are easily recognizable by their gaits.
Since no one's feet match anyone else's, individual gaits abound.
Nearsighted folk report that, without glasses, they use gait as a

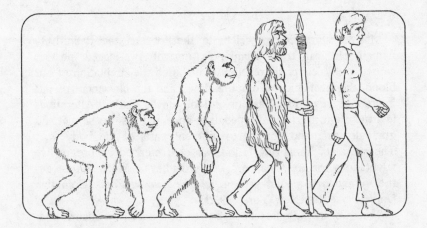

point of recognition when looking for someone in a crowd. After all, we may mistake someone by hair color or clothing, but how they walk is generally an unchanging factor. This explains why "normal" gait includes a fairly wide range of patterns. Foot doctors are not dealing with one ideal means of locomotion but rather with a large range of variation in theoretically acceptable stances. However, once we step out of these bounds, problems will manifest themselves. And not necessarily only in our feet: our knees and spinal columns will feel the brunt if our feet are not working properly. As long as our weight is transmitted from the heel along the foot's outer edge to the ball and finally to the big toe, we're on the right path. Examine the soles of your shoes for clues to your own walking habits.

Without a doubt, we have made enormous strides since prehistoric times when we straightened up from a bridgelike position and threw all our weight onto our two feet. This metamorphosis meant a shift in the body's center of gravity that involved adjustments in all the body's joints, particularly in the spine. In the upright posture, the vertebrae became more susceptible to the impact conveyed upward with each step; intervertebral disks acted as buffers to soften the blows. Heels and arches appeared in our feet in order to aid in forward motion; knees and hips also took on new duties as muscles adjusted to keeping us vertical and in action.

Many anthropologists celebrate the foot as the definitively human physical trait. Mankind's upright two-legged posture caused a physical chain reaction that shifted the circulation of our blood, the mechanics of our breathing, and the placement of our internal organs, as well as our outlook on the world. "Alterations in structure for terrestrial bipedalism appeared first in the feet and gradually extended upward to different parts of the body . . . The course of human evolution was characterized by progressive adaptations for erect stance," writes Dudley J. Morton, foot authority and orthopedic surgeon, in *The Human Foot* (Columbia University Press, New York, 1935).

Traces of evolutionary changes can be detected in such a phenomenon as the so-called Grecian foot, distinguished by a second toe that extends farther than the big toe, a holdover from an earlier stage of mankind's development. Gradually the formerly thumb-like big toe, which has fallen into the same plane as the others, will overpower all of them. The heel, which now rests on the ground to support body weight better, and the arches contribute to the stride we take for granted. Adaptive measures like these are regarded by anthropologists as the most significant in the history of evolution.

By the transfer of the locomotive process to the lower extremities, the rest of the body was free to perform other tasks. It is really to our feet that we owe our humanness. As Duke University anthropologist Weston La Barre wrote: "Man stands alone because he alone stands."

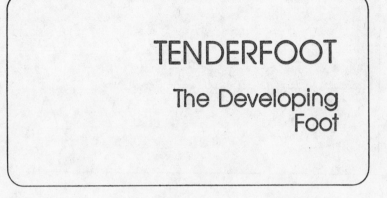

# TENDERFOOT
## The Developing Foot

The infant foot is strikingly reminiscent of our anthropoidal fore-fathers: its toes possess twenty times the grip strength of its adult counterpart and it is capable of functions normally associated with the hand. The foot and leg appear in the fetus by the sixth week of human pregnancy and then double in size in the fifth month. Except for an occasional poke, the feet are at rest in the womb. The fetus, however, is curled up and this position will later affect the infant's body configuration, according to Dr. Richard Schuster. "Since we lie on one side in the womb, we tend to favor this side later on," he claims. And just as most of us will become right-handed, most of us become right-footed—a possible clue as to why there is a predominance of people with shorter left legs.

A baby's foot consists of as much soft tissue as bone although this bone is still soft. "The bones are soft and pliant in the fetus and they stay that way for a longer time than most people realize. The properly straightened foot does not finish growing until about age twenty," Dr. Schuster says. In fact, the infant foot has fewer bones than the adult since they have not yet calcified; in this

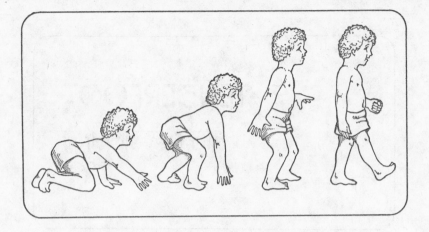

fibrous state, they don't register on X-rays. By adult standards, the normal infant foot appears unfamiliar in its softness. An average newborn's foot is 3 to 3¼ inches long and will grow to about 9 inches in the average adult female and about 11 inches in the average adult male. Although the baby foot may seem unusual to the adult eye, it may be the ideal of a "normal" foot since no calluses or corns have had time to develop. It's only a matter of time before all irregularities that afflict the defenseless adult foot begin to emerge.

The long arch, hidden beneath a layer of fat until about age three, is unprepared for any strain during the first six months of life. From both aesthetic and superstitious points of view, flatfeet are viewed as stigmas and thereby a cause for widespread parental concern. But until the fat pad abates and the adult foot emerges, there is no reason for a parent to worry. If flat-footedness is a family trait, there is a greater chance your baby will inherit a flat but serviceable foot and will never suffer the discomfort of a fallen arch. To check for signs of good foot health, look for the alignments of the growing child's foot with the leg, toes with the foot, and knees with the foot. You can do this before you diaper the baby by laying it on its stomach. Then check to see that the creases under the buttocks are symmetrical. Should one buttock appear flatter or wider, consult your pediatrician. Unless one of these alignments seems unnatural, don't worry. If an imbalance exists, your doctor will prescribe proper measures.

Any stress on the foot during infancy could have permanent repercussions: ligaments may stretch out of shape and bones may be thrown out of alignment. So as a rule, don't constrict your baby's foot. Avoid shoes or even booties. This need for foot freedom applies to any foot covering for a child; blankets should be loosely wrapped and socks should be roomy and not of the stretch variety that might distort toes. In order to guarantee your child's proper foot development, watch out for three adverse circumstances: improper sleeping postures, premature weight bearing, and hard surfaces.

Crib position can make a big difference in foot growth. A baby's lying face down encourages toenails to curl into the toes. The nails will grow out eventually, but the parent can avoid this complication by turning the baby as it sleeps. Keep in mind that the foot is an organ comprising bones, muscles, and tendons which require use to develop correctly. Flexing the toes is a form of exercise which is prevented if baby lies in one position only in the crib.

If your baby prefers to sleep on its side in the fetal position, avoid cramping of the feet by propping the baby from behind with a rolled blanket or placing the blanket along the front of its torso, since the baby's body is not yet strong enough to roll onto its back.

Parents eager to see their babies walking may risk improper development by lifting the infant onto its feet. Holding the baby up may strain unprepared muscles, and this premature weight bearing can lead to later complications such as bowleggedness.

Until the baby is able to walk unaided, the best place to practice upright posture is on a pliant surface. The playpen is the usual site of such experimentation. By covering the thin mattress with a soft blanket, the baby's feet will stay warm while its toes will flex against the soft material and build strength.

When the baby feels ready to stand, that miracle will occur. But until the moment arrives, it is foolish to push the child. Parental pride may rush the natural course of events, but "helping" the process along may harm the musculature of the foot and leg. Use of a walker (a self-propelled chair) is not recommended until the child is able to walk, since this practice tends to put the wrong stress on muscles and create the same type of pressure on feet as do high heels on adult women. Naturally, the heavier baby may be more hesitant to rely on wobbly legs and may wait it out a bit longer. Cute as the baby looks standing, its feet will pay for it later if they are not prepared for the task.

The first year of life is generally considered the most important period of physical development for the foot since it is pliable and the growth rate is rapid. By the time a baby reaches its first birthday, its feet should have attained half their adult size; full growth will be completed by a person's twenty-first year.

Years ago doctors treated children like small adults, but soon they came to realize that until age twelve, every age group—separated by two-year intervals—has different problems. New examination techniques were developed to accommodate each stage of growth. For your own information, the podiatrist Dr. Elizabeth Roberts suggests the following timetable:

 6 months—crawls, little use of the feet.
 8 months—tries to stand.
12 months—stands well.
14 months—walks without aid.
18 months—walks well.
24 months—runs.
36 months—runs and jumps.

This guide gives you an *approximate* idea as to what to expect; however, since there is no exact age at which specific progress occurs, don't panic if your child doesn't conform. After all, little Albert Einstein didn't start talking until age three!

For best results in your baby's development, follow these simple rules:

1  Avoid socks and shoes unless absolutely necessary for warmth. Apply the same principle as for the hands—they don't *always* have to be covered against the elements.

2 Allow the baby to be uncovered indoors for a certain amount of time each day so that it can kick without interference. Naturally, there must be adequate heat to ensure that the baby will not catch cold.

3 Always check to see that footwear is sufficiently roomy; this might mean larger sock sizes every six weeks or so.

4 Move the baby from the stomach position to the back to give different muscles the opportunity to flex.

5 Cut toenails straight across at the tips of the toes to avoid ingrown nails or accidental scratching.

Most problems that occur in these early years are outgrown in time. As the old saying reminds us: "Nature cures the illness, but the doctor gets the fee." As the baby plays with its feet, toe muscles flex and develop. Shoes may interfere with the natural course of events. Even once baby is toddling, shoes are not necessary indoors; muscles will develop more fully on their own. Out in the real world of concrete, however, footgear is required.

Until the baby's body has found its center of gravity, apparent imbalances may arise. Limping may simply indicate temporary favoritism of one leg over the other. While the feet begin to develop strength, the baby's walk is characteristically unsteady. If there is an obvious limp, look for underlying causes: cuts, jagged toenails, warts, blisters. In school-age children, a syndrome commonly known as the "ten-day limp" occurs for no apparent reason and disappears just as mysteriously, as if on cue.

Toeing in or out may persist even once the child's feet are more or less parallel during walking. "Pigeon toes" should not alarm you; this is another part of the growth process and should resolve itself in time. Toddlers tend to toe in at first to maintain balance. Between the ages of one and a half and three, the child's walking patterns should be medically checked during the routine visit to your pediatrician. If the situation prevails after age three, your doctor can advise further measures to take.

"Pronation" refers to toeing out à la Charlie Chaplin. This causes the longitudinal arch to flatten as muscles weaken, especially those muscles at the subtalar joint near the ankle. Exercises

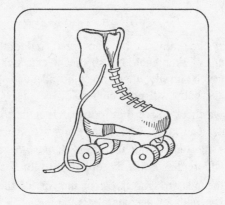

may be the answer or a splint may be needed to correct this abnormality if it is not outgrown. Until age six, most of the child's foot problems can be considered temporary. After this turning point, the U. S. Public Health Service estimates that 87 per cent of Americans will suffer from some type of foot affliction.

Although most children visit pediatricians on a regular basis, their feet are often overlooked. Many podiatrists point out that during routine checkups, doctors often neglect to remove a child's socks. Feet, just like any other part of the body, must be examined for proper development, but many pediatricians' exams don't go below the knee where harmful shoes or foot infections may be having a field day.

Ideally, we should spend the first six or seven years of our lives barefoot. Once shoes enter the picture, a whole new spectrum of complications is introduced. First of all, the rate of foot growth is still so rapid that shoe size may get larger every month or two. While sneakers were formerly dismissed as unsuitable for everyday wear, at present they are lauded as the best footwear for children. Sneakers have skyrocketed in popularity since 1957 when they only represented 10 per cent of the entire shoe market. "No support" was the catchphrase used to condemn their nonleather structure. Today they account for 50 per cent of shoes sold domestically. Clearly, the days of taboo are over. Any podiatrist will tell you that sneakers are congenial footwear; some even admit that they don't allow their children to wear any other shoe, which is convenient, since sneakers are now fashionable among the younger set. Yes, podiatrists will go so far as to say that they love sneakers! The only drawback concerns foot hygiene: the rubber binding and sole tend to attract moisture and heat, creating a welcome environment for certain kinds of fungus. But as long as feet are washed regularly, sneakers should pose no problem.

The days of "corrective" shoes are over, too. Didn't you ever as a child secretly question the purpose of clomping around in those unattractive, heavy shoes? Not to mention their social stigma among your peers! Those were the days when we ogled our loafer-shod elders enviously. Instead, we were weighted down in black lace-ups—which are conspicuously absent in children's wardrobes nowadays. Enough is enough! With luck, your feet have recovered since then and you are now prancing nimbly through the years. Today sneakers are suggested as a corrective means to improve a child's gait. Rigid so-called corrective footwear only serves to aggravate juvenile foot problems in most cases, especially those which involve toeing in or out. Even ordinary children's footwear is often too heavy or "grown up" and can consequently hamper normal gait. Walking barefoot would be the solution for children, allowing for any irregularity to adjust itself. But since circumstances usually prevent romping unshod, wearing sneakers is the next best thing.

"Ankle support" is another dead issue. The normal ankle should support itself. Dr. Roberts sees only a single advantage to high-laced shoes for a baby: they are harder to remove and lose. Otherwise, the child's ankle will do fine on its own rather than with artificial help. Low shoes are also cooler and should provide all the necessary support. Nothing is wrong with sandals, either, which allow free toe movement. Educated medical opinion agrees with the American Indian that the all-purpose moccasin is an ideal shoe for the tot.

Flexibility is the key to good shoes. For fitting shoes, the child should be standing. Shoes should be about ½ inch longer than the longest toe. Look for snug heel fit; tie shoes are preferable since they can be adjusted to hug the heel—loafers slip off too easily. Hand-me-down shoes for children will probably mean hand-me-down problems later; also resoling their shoes may mean compromising the integrity of the shoe fit—since feet grow so quickly at this age, it may be just as well to invest in a new pair.

Parents must be on their toes to ensure their child's better foot health, particularly since children may be reticent about expressing discomfort. Signs to watch for: shoes that bulge at the inner ankle, or that roll toward the outside, the constant removal of shoes, irregular walking habits, or shoes that wear out at the tips.

Another clue would be "growing pains" in the legs. Rather than growth, such pains indicate lack of oxygen in the muscles, which might be a possible side effect of improper foot balance. Or the pains might indicate sore muscles due to overactivity which a simple massage can cure. Check the relationship of the child's buttocks to the foot for hip deficiency; there may be a congenital dislocation. If you have any doubts, your pediatrician will give you the answers.

There are basically three complaints that occur exclusively in children, and although these are not widespread, parents should be aware of their symptoms. The natural growing process of bone may sometimes "compete" for the blood supply. Until the circulation is stabilized, there may be some pain. One example of this temporary discomfort is Köhler's bone disease, prevalent among the three-to-eight-year age group. It is a degeneration of the navicular bone. Pains near the longitudinal arch, as well as a possible swelling in that area, will signal its presence. Resting the foot and arch supports (rubber "cookies") will provide relief until the blood supply catches up with bone growth.

Freiberg's infraction also involves bone degeneration, this time of the head of the second metatarsal bone. Although growth may also be responsible here, injury to the second toe may contribute to this type of hairline fracture. Again, rest, with the help of a metatarsal pad, will do the trick.

As the child approaches adolescence, the third complaint may arise—an aching heel. This usually happens when the Achilles tendon gets inflamed; the condition is known as "adolescent calcaneodynia (*calcaneus:* heel; *-odynia:* pain), or, more commonly, "growing pains." Pressure of any kind aggravates the condition, which may afflict one or both feet. Attaching a ½-inch lift into the shoe heel will ease the tension ordinarily placed upon the Achilles tendon; this generally solves the problem.

In general, the best way for us to prevent those foot problems we can control is to promote good hygiene habits in our children. Where internal disorders are concerned, parents should be aware of warning signals such as limping or excessive pain. Once children begin to bathe themselves, they should learn to blot their feet dry, especially between the toes. In this way, fungal infections can be averted. Barefooted frolicking should be confined to the home, the beach, and the sandbox; after all, those little "piggies" have a long road ahead of them.

# FOOTPRINTS IN THE SAND
## Foot Types

*"Feet are as variable as faces."*
DR. RICHARD SCHUSTER

Although we all hope to start out on the right foot, some circumstances are completely out of our control. By accident of birth, we are subject to genetic variations or even deformities in our feet. To these we have to add the man-made variations that result from the crazy things we make our feet do. The combination of these elements creates a large variety of diverse foot types.

For clues about how each of us get our particular pair of feet, we have to inspect our genes. Hereditary factors determine whether we will sport the tapered Grecian foot with a longer second toe or the wide forefoot with narrow heel so common among women. The "Greek" foot, a term derived from ancient mythology, as noted above, originally referred to those goddesses with longer second toes, symbolic of their special male powers. Although dancers on pointe may regret having the Grecian-foot configuration, there should be no other reason for complaint. A few people inherit webbed toes, a genetic anomaly when a membrane

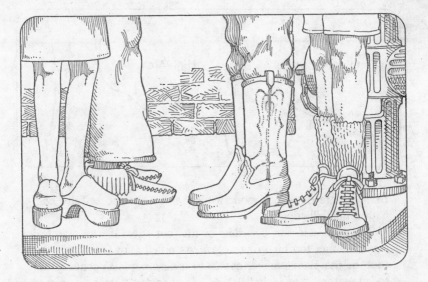

connects (usually) the second and third toes. Again, this does not affect walking and is altogether harmless.

Feet may tilt in any direction due to weak muscles or incorrect alignment. The foot that turns upward so that the first toe seems to be on a higher plane is known as "forefoot varus." Conversely, the foot in which the little toe tilts upward is called "forefoot valgus." As for the heel, when turned outward, it is a "heel varus," when turned inward, a "heel valgus."

Many children are born with foot abnormalities due to improper positions in the uterus. These problems can be easily corrected at birth; the obstetrician simply adjusts the foot by "passive overcorrection," or manually adjusting the position of the foot so that it will then self-regulate. A clubfoot, or talipes, is treated in this manner. Most often the clubfoot is bent down and inward so that walking would involve only the toes and the outside of the foot. Sometimes the foot bends up and outward, which means that the heel is the only point of contact with the ground. Treatment can begin one week after birth—massage, manipulation and casts can correct the malleable infant foot. In extreme cases, surgery may be required. But certainly the agonies of the clubfooted intern described by W. Somerset Maugham in his 1915 novel *Of Human*

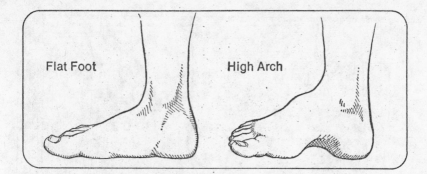

Flat Foot        High Arch

*Bondage* are outdated; modern technology has successfully combatted this affliction.

The most common disorders of the foot affect the long arch; it may be either too high or too low. As noted above, a child's flatfoot, or pes planus, never ceases to arouse parental concern. But today, natural, congenital flatfeet are considered strong and serviceable foundations. In the past, the United States Army routinely rejected flatfooted men even before determining whether the condition was congenital or acquired. Actually, people with congenital flatfeet are well-suited to marching, in contrast to those with higher arched feet that might collapse under rigorous strain. (The Army has since revised its policy.)

When not congenital, flatfeet can often be identified if the ankles lean toward each other. This means that the subtalar joint (beneath the ankle) is out of order and so a weak ankle results. Or, because of a series of injuries or improper walking habits, the ligaments in the foot may literally collapse. Rather than carrying on their duty as keepers of the foot, the ligaments may lose control. The foot then spreads, to become ever more square-shaped. Fatigue, especially at the end of the day, and pain, ranging from a sore arch to aches reaching up to the knee, are the hallmarks of the fallen arch. Discomfort may also attack other parts of the body: the spine becomes more vulnerable since the foot is no longer a shock absorber and so impacts reverberate upward with more force.

Consider the following questions if you want to check yourself for flatfeet: Do your stiff and sore feet ease up after you pad about in the morning? Does the pain peak in the early afternoon? Do you look forward with great anticipation to kicking off your shoes at night? Foot strain manifests itself similarly, but if pain persists or worsens, only a doctor will be able to help. Supportive devices or surgery—a last resort—will prevent total collapse.

On the other hand, the high arch, or pes cavus, is equally troublesome but tends to be transmitted genetically. Usually, the high-arched foot only requires well-fitted shoes or metatarsal arch supports to correct the weight-bearing pattern. The heads of the metatarsals may ache due to the shape of the foot, and calluses may then develop since so much pressure is exerted on that area. As long as you don't force your high-arched foot to lean on the inner sole, they should cause you no pain *if* the shoe fits.

An extremely high arch may curl the toes under in a configuration known as a "clawfoot." In severe cases, where it is due to cerebral palsy or polio, the muscles may be badly damaged. These instances require surgical correction.

Another common variety of foot shape concerns the toes. A child's "pigeon toes" may cause much parental anxiety, undue since the condition is often outgrown. If they are hereditary because of hip formation, a parent's awareness even before the child walks will reduce the problem considerably. Stretching exercises will help the child's muscles to develop correctly; in most cases the turned-in stance will then disappear.

Although time is the great healer, we can improve our chances for proper gait by taking care of our feet. Unlike days of yore, we can now overcome many of the irregularities in our walking patterns that cause discomfort by combining medical attention with tender loving care.

# FOOT IMPRESSIONS
## Myths and Superstitions

*"The head and feet keep warm—*
*The rest will take no harm."*
ANONYMOUS

Fascination with the foot dates back before biblical times. Achilles' heel as described in mythology still stands as the precursor of heel pain (and point of vulnerability) through the ages. As the story goes, while dipping him in waters said to make him invulnerable, Achilles' mother held him by one heel—an oversight for which he probably never forgave her. He later lost his life in the Trojan War when a well-placed poisoned arrow found his heel.

Starting off on the "right foot" meant the one on the right side in ancient Rome. Romans believed the gods resided in the right side of the body, which was therefore impervious to tumultuous emotions. Special "footmen" were employed by noblemen to check which foot the guests entered upon; these duties changed in later times. Shakespeare echoed this ritual in *Titus Andronicus:* "Come on, my lords, the better foot before." Seafaring folk carry this ancient tradition into the present day by stepping with the right foot onto the deck of a ship making its maiden voyage.

The imprint of the foot can have awesome connotations. From the 3½-million-year-old footprints found by anthropologist Mary Leakey in Tanzania to Neil Armstrong's first step on the moon, the footprint has gathered quite a reputation. The footprint in certain cultures is considered an extension of the personality. Some Australian Aborigine tribes "cripple" their enemies by stabbing sharp objects into their footprints. Leaving a distinct footprint behind may be asking for trouble in some parts of the world. In former days in Bohemia, one way to lame an adversary was to boil the earth of his footprint with a nail, a needle, and some broken glass until the kettle cracks. Estonians preferred to measure the footprint with a stick and then bury that part of the stick for sure results.

In Burma and Northern India sores on the foot are often attributed to footprint voodoo. Many African tribes cover their tracks and bless scuttling insects that help obliterate them and thus prevent evil interference. And then there are Bigfoot, or Sasquatch, in the Northwest United States, and the Abominable Snowman, or Yeti, in the Himalayas who leave marks wherever they roam. The latter mythical monster can be recognized only by his oversized footprints since few have laid eyes on him. The skeptics explain the impressions as a large bear's pawprints, but this is merely speculation.

Footprints also serve as a love charm. Zuñi Indian women guard their husbands' footprints in order to keep them faithful. And, if accidentally found, the footprint of the Egyptian goddess Isis was said to banish infertility. Of course, it may be difficult to recognize a supernatural footprint as in the case of Adam's Peak in Sri Lanka. This large rock, which bears a depression in the shape of a footprint, has become the site of religious pilgrimages by people of different faiths. Muslims believe that it is the mark of Adam, Buddhists recognize it as the sacred footstep of Buddha, while Hindus view it as that of Siva.

Foot kissing evolved out of an Asian custom of obeisance. It became a gesture of submission toward a person of lofty stature: a king, pope, or saint. Eventually the gesture disappeared, with the exception of the kissing of the embroidered cross on the pontifical shoe, a religious rather than a servile action. Foot washing caught on in commemoration of Christ's washing the feet of the apostles at the Last Supper. The Egyptians always bathed their feet before each meal and even applied perfume to them.

The removal of shoes at the threshold of a holy place is observed by Muslims, Hindus, and Buddhists alike. This custom also is mentioned in Exodus when God instructs Moses to "Put off thy shoes from off thy feet, for the place whereon thou standest is holy ground."

Holding one's shoes has been interpreted as an assertive act. In the Psalms, the phrase "Over Edom I cast out my shoe" implies that one can claim land by planting one's foot on it.

Shoes and feet have traditionally played a starring role in marriage rituals. Feet seem to be the universal symbol of the male genitalia, a phallic symbol. Foot length has been a traditionally delicate subject since it is often considered indicative of genital size. In 1826 Sir Walter Scott wrote: "I think I know the length of that man's foot; we have had a jollification or so together." And if size means anything, the old woman who lived in a shoe was undeniably oversexed.

In the realm of courtship, feet and their adjuncts participate in its rituals around the world. In biblical times, Hebrew swains presented their fiancées with a shoe as well as a ring to symbolize mutual possession of worldly goods. Tying shoes to the car of a newlywed couple today is the vestige of an ancient custom symbolizing the bride's walking away from the parental hearth. French tradition dictated that the bride keep her wedding shoes as a guarantee that the union will last happily ever after. Sicilian girls of yore would keep a shoe under their pillows at night to help the search for husbands. An early American custom required a hopeful young lady to place her shoes beside the bed with the heel of one against the middle of the other shoe in a tau (Greek T) configuration, a symbol of fertility; this would then ensure sweet dreams and happiness in love.

On the Eve of St. Andreas—the German patron saint of lovers—unmarried girls used to increase their chances of finding a suitable partner with whom to have a large family by rubbing their feet against the bedpost. (For Slavs, St. Lucia serves the same purpose and is the proper source to whom to address one's heartaches.) After marriage, one superstition holds that getting out of bed should be done with both feet at once in order to avert bad luck.

"May you fit her as this old shoe has fit her," goes an old Anglo-Saxon marriage toast. Then the bride's father presents his daughter's shoe to the groom in a symbolic transferral of authority. To prove her domestic talents, the new bride may now choose to challenge the old English proverb: "The foot on the cradle and hand on the distaff is the sign of a good housewife." This statement was spoken upon entering a room where a woman was spinning while rocking the baby's cradle with her foot.

Divorce among Arabs was readily available by the ritual which required the husband to place his wife's shoes outdoors and announce: "She has been my slipper; I cast her out now!" Using the same metaphor, a Roman explaining his divorce asked: "Is not my shoe handsome and new? But no one of you can tell me where it pinches me."

For the Chinese, the woman's foot was once the ultimate sex symbol—if it conformed to the ideal "lilylike" structure. From the eleventh century until the early twentieth this meant the binding of the females' feet in order to prevent the bones from developing in the usual way. Stunting foot growth would result in the desired shape, making the foot the most attractive part of the female anatomy. This custom allegedly began as a result of Empress Taki's clubfoot; an edict forced all women to bind their feet in a way simulating this distortion, starting this age-old fad.

Lovemaking in old China included plenty of attention to the delicate lotus foot for the ultimate sensual experience. Pornography regarding the feet abounded. The mere sight of an exposed bound foot was enough to set a man's imagination aflame. Since Confucius' time, a woman's small foot was extolled as the most lovely of all her physical traits. The shrinking process involved bringing the front and rear of the foot toward each other, halving the natural size. Plumpness, softness, and fineness could then be cultivated to add to the essential attraction.

Creating a Chinese woman's lotus feet was a long process which

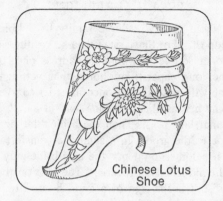

Chinese Lotus
Shoe

started at age five or so. The feet were bound and with each passing year, the bandages tightened as the bones became more rigid.
Knowing how desirable she would finally become provided
sufficient motivation and dulled any discomfort—not unlike the
motivation behind wearing high heels in the modern Western
world. Peer pressure would prevent any dissent. By her teen years,
the young girl would have mastered the art of wrapping the 10-
foot-long bandage around her own feet. Western influence soon
put an end to this uniquely Oriental custom and in 1902 a decree
made foot binding in China illegal—although it could never outlaw
the inherent allure of the feet.

Attitudes toward feet manifest in imaginative ways in different
cultures. In Japan, many people choose to sleep with their feet on
the pillow. Doctors agree with this practice as an efficient means
of improving circulation. An old German custom involved placing
a pair of shoes—heels outward—at the head of the bed to ward off
nightmares. Disappointed Englishmen used to say, "You have
made a hand into a foot," to express discontent.

For good luck, colonial Americans used to spit into their right
shoe before putting it on; this custom had also been common in
Roman times—presumably as effective as talc.

Stumbling is a traditional sign of foreboding. Ancient belief
held that tripping over a threshold when entering a house was an
omen that the visitor was untrustworthy, imbued with evil powers.
To undo this bad luck, the old formula "I turn myself around
three times about, and thus I put bad luck to rout" was believed to
work. Snapping your fingers was also claimed to be an efficient

means of dispelling evil spirits. The greatest fear in stumbling was that the all-too-loosely hinged human soul might slip out, never to return. On the other hand, stumbling into your own house was a good sign from which we derive the expression "I fell into it," meaning "I had an accidental piece of luck."

To add to your Monday-morning blues, one Old English adage warned, "It is unlucky to meet a man with flatfeet on a Monday morning." Fortunately, this curse could be reversed by returning home, eating and drinking and setting out again—on the right foot.

If you intend to have a New Year's party, remember the Northumberland saying that "Good luck for a year will accrue to a house entered on New Year's morning by a person with a high instep." An old British custom—"firstfooting"—was, and in Scotland still is, commonly practiced after the New Year arrives. Friends and neighbors are expected to visit each other—signifying what the future has in store. One biased saying claims that, "It will bring bad luck to the house for a year if the first person to cross the threshold on New Year's Day is a woman." Omens of good luck vary with the region. In general, if the "firstfooter" is a dark-haired man, all will be well. Originally, firstfooters used to bring a present of a shovelful of coal—now they bring a bottle of Scotch.

No matter how you tread, superstition has made it difficult not to put one's foot in one's mouth. Watching your step can be serious business.

# BATTERED FEET

Battered feet—a hush-hush topic often covered up by its worst offenders. Why is no one willing to discuss the crimes that occur within the confines of a shoe? We speak of our feet "killing" us as if they had devised an intelligent plan of attack which we can never hope to combat. Yet we insist upon cramping them into tight, pointy shoes, secretly wishing that they will suffocate and our pains will be over forever!

No such luck. As we seem to forget, our feet are very much the foundation upon which we try to stand—sometimes as off center as the Leaning Tower of Pisa. When they begin to ache, this usually means that they are not properly supporting the rest of our body. And when they're not doing their job, the rest of the body is thrown out of kilter. Without our feet taking the brunt of each step, the impact is felt up to the spine and may cause serious damage. The sooner we come to terms with our feet, the sooner our suffering will end. "The only real hope of eliminating foot problems is to spend your whole life walking barefoot on a sandy beach," says Dr. Suzanne Levine of Mt. Sinai Hospital and the

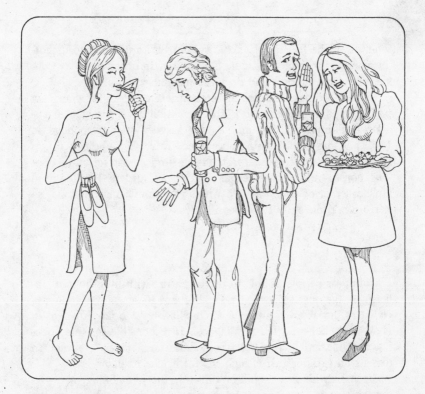

Yorkville Foot Center in New York City. But short of beachcombing in the tropical climes, we can at least educate ourselves on the nature of our feet and gain the upper hand in the struggle to walk happily.

Any variation in the leg structure has its final expression in the foot. Stabilization is possible with modern techniques. Biomechanics is a new branch of medical engineering concerned with the dynamics of human motion. By studying the range of normal/abnormal motion, doctors are able to adjust footfall and eliminate pain with the help of custom-made "orthotics." These devices—formerly called "foot appliances," "inserts," "plates," "arch supports"—do not work on the principle of supporting the arches. Instead, the relationship of each part of the foot to the surface underfoot is analyzed; orthotics are then designed to improve the function of the feet and legs. "Post controls" are added to orthotics wherever a change in angle is necessary in order to better control abnormal motion and decrease instability.

Even if orthotics are not the appropriate antidote for your foot problem, pain-free walking is still a possibility. A big step in podiatry—minimal incision ambulatory surgery—was introduced in 1962 and has been gaining acceptance rapidly. Pinhole incisions replace their larger counterparts in the surgical correction of bunions, corns, and hammertoes, among other disorders. Hurting need not be a fact of everyday life with these simple new options, so step up and check out the possibilities.

# Arthritis

Countless people hobble to the podiatrist with little hope of relief from the onset of arthritis. Dr. Bernard Rosenstein, a foot specialist at the arthritis clinic at Columbia-Presbyterian Hospital in New York, believes that misdiagnosis is responsible for this hopeless attitude and that relief is a definite possibility. "I straighten toes as an orthodontist straightens teeth," he explains.

Since arthritis is a condition affecting the joint lining, it favors the large network of bones in the feet. Arthritis results when the spaces between the metatarsals increase or decrease, causing pain; or sometimes spicules—small, needle-shaped particles—may develop and create arthritic conditions. Further discomfort results from poor alignment of the feet with the rest of the body, which will have a chain-reaction effect by aggravating symptoms of arthritis that were hitherto in a latent form.

To be able to deal effectively with arthritis, you must discern which of the three forms you have: gout, osteoarthritis, or rheumatoid arthritis.

## GOUT

An excess of uric acid in the body, due to faulty kidney function, may build up in the joint spaces as the result of faulty internal protein processing. When the body has a hard time metabolizing purines—compounds found in such foods as anchovies, sardines, other small fish, and organ meats—gout will flare up. Although there is no solid proof, it is believed to be a hereditary disorder; unofficial statistics claim that 10 to 20 per cent of all gout victims have other gout sufferers among their relatives. Excess purine in the blood is indicated by the uric acid crystals it produces; these crystals can be found most commonly in the ear lobes, feet, elbows, knees, and wrists. If you have gout, you can often feel lumps of this chalky deposit in your ear lobes. When these deposits settle in the big toe, which then becomes inflamed, the pain may be crippling. Even the mere weight of a bed sheet will send a deeply painful sensation through the foot; chills, fever, or rapid heartbeat may accompany the inflammation.

Gout attacks generally favor the big toe, which then turns deep red and swells. A particularly stressful, emotionally draining event or a meal high in purine usually precedes a gout attack. Medical attention is imperative in order to control swelling. A single blood test will confirm whether it is gout. The earlier the condition is recognized, the better it will respond to medication and tissue damage can be kept to a minimum.

Gout is a chronic disease which only shows its true colors in the acute phase. Recurrence is inevitable if correct steps are not taken. Lifelong medication will regulate the amount of uric acid in the bloodstream and avert further attacks. Of the three types of arthritis, it is the only one that can be controlled.

Contrary to popular myth, gout is not an affliction exclusive to the idle dandy. Rather, the disease is most prevalent among highly intelligent and ambitious men; in fact, gout is a sort of perverse status symbol. Since Egyptian times, this excruciating condition has been chronicled in cartoons and caricatures. Hippocrates in the fifth century B.C. dubbed it "the unwalkable disease" and remarked that "eunuchs do not take the gout [and] young men do not either until they indulge in coition." Of the 1 million Americans suffering of gout, 95 per cent are male; the remaining 5 per cent consists mainly, for reasons as yet unknown, of women who have passed menopause.

Famous gout victims have allegedly been Achilles, Oedipus, Kublai Khan, Erasmus, Michelangelo, and Leonardo da Vinci. John Milton was said to have been inspired by gout when he wrote about Hell in *Paradise Lost*. Among English royal victims, James I and Henry VIII can be counted; Henry VI was obliged to postpone his wedding because of this unpredictable ailment.

Although there is no cure per se for gout, several drug programs have been designed to prevent future onslaughts. Unfortunately, the side effects of drugs may be equally distracting, so a bit of experimentation, under your doctor's guidance, will help you find which one works best for you. Colchicine heads the list and has been an antidote since ancient Egyptian days. However, an upset stomach may be the price for getting rid of gout this way. Phenylbutazone (an anti-inflammatory), probenecid (which increases the excretion of uric acid by the kidneys), and allopurinol (which reduces the production of uric acid by the kidneys) each combat gout from different angles. Cortisone injections may relieve symptoms without restoring health, whereas a posterior nerve block injection will force blood into the foot while flushing out the uric crystals.

During a gout attack, rest is necessary—and will be the victim's instinctive reaction—in order to keep body weight off the joints. Drinking water in large amounts (up to 3 quarts per day) will dilute the urate (uric acid salts) in the kidneys.

Although medical opinion is mixed as to whether a regulated diet will help to prevent further gout attacks, it is probably advisable for the sufferer to avoid foods high in purine content. Alcohol should also be kept to a minimum. Suggested foods include soybeans, lima beans, potatoes, and bananas. Also "cherry therapy" is highly recommended and the fruit should be taken on a daily basis as a sort of natural "pill." Cherries are helpful in any form since they react in the body to control uric acid levels in the blood.

## OSTEOARTHRITIS

Over the years, walking, running, repeated injuries, and ill-fitting shoes all take their toll on those innocent bystanders, the feet. Microtraumas accumulate and then, one day, arthritis appears. Natural wear and tear finally overcomes all systems, and, being low men on the totem pole, your feet are more vulnerable to this abuse than are other parts of the body.

Eroded cartilage around the joints, changing joint shape, and weak muscles all attest to permanent damage caused by the combination of foot imbalance and the natural deterioration of the skeleton after age twenty-five. Overweight adds to the burden already hoisted upon those weatherbeaten tootsies—weight, at least, can be controlled and will make a big difference down there. Since your feet are more sensitive once they begin to degenerate, small things you never thought about before may irritate an arthritic area. For example, if you lace your shoes too tightly, irritation under the laces may result. If this should happen, soak your feet until discomfort abates.

The anti-inflammatory components of aspirin should also ease arthritic pain. The American Medical Association (AMA) recommends twelve to twenty 5-grain tablets per day; if aspirin is not strong enough, ask your doctor to suggest something else. Corrective aids such as Dr. Rosenstein's "toe sleeves" should also help to relieve discomfort. These aids work like an orthodontist's retainer device on teeth braces by gradually bringing the toes into the proper position. It may take six months to one year for there to be any appreciable movement, but the patient's discomfort is usually relieved immediately. More than 90 per cent of Dr. Rosenstein's arthritis patients have been able to avoid surgery and improve their condition in this way.

In more advanced cases, surgery may be the only solution. Scraping the joint clean or providing artificial replacements are two common methods used by surgeons. "Toe implants" are gaining in popularity since their appearance in 1967. In this procedure, one of the joints of the big toe is surgically removed and replaced by a prosthetic implant: half-joints, spacers, or hinged devices may be used. The artificial implant will maintain the correct toe alignment without the possibility of erosion. The University of California Medical Center in Los Angeles showed that of their first nineteen patients undergoing this procedure, the majority have regained the ability to walk. These implants restore flexibility in the big toe which is integral to "toeing off" when you walk and shift all your weight onto that joint.

## Rheumatoid Arthritis

Unlike the other two forms of arthritis, which are confined to people over twenty-five, rheumatoid arthritis of the feet has no age limit, nor is it hereditary. Children can be afflicted with this condition and suffer permanent damage. Sometimes, rheumatic fever may be responsible for it, as a secondary infection. Otherwise, there is no known cause. The victim may have no history of foot disorders preceding its onslaught—a sudden bump may occur one day without warning and develop into rheumatoid arthritis. It strikes acutely at intervals, but is always present in a latent state. Fever, fatigue, and loss of appetite are the warning signals which precede an attack, as well as swelling in the finger and toe joints and a tingling sensation in the feet.

Rheumatoid arthritis is three times more common among women than among men, although there is no known reason as to why this is. It can be easily recognized by the distortion of the toes which veer off at unnatural angles. Heberden's nodes, or bony protuberances, may appear over the end of the joint. Or bunions that deform the foot to an extreme degree may appear. And when it spreads, rheumatoid arthritis can be a crippler.

Emotional stress has been known to trigger this condition—as if the foot is signaling that it literally cannot stand whatever is going on. Although there is no definitive medical explanation of how the emotions trigger reactions in the feet, research is under way in an effort to determine their power. On the other hand, Dr. Rosenstein's experience leads him to believe that a virus is at the root of this condition, a virus which might easily be tamed once identified. Definitive results remain to be seen in both cases.

Again, aspirin is a main combatant of rheumatoid arthritis. Unless immediate measures are taken to harness this disorder, inflammation may spread through the connective body tissues. However, rheumatoid arthritis has an unpredictable life-span and may burn out after a while, leaving a trail of permanent damage but releasing its victim from acute agonies.

Although the podiatrist may not be able to "cure" arthritis, he or she can take mechanical measures to ease the situation. Before

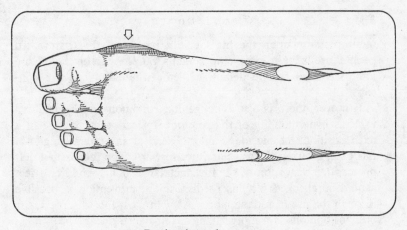

Bunion in early stages.

foot problems grow to this magnitude, see a rheumatologist. Your main concern should be to keep moving and keep on your feet—while it is still in your power.

## Bunions

Thanks to evolutionary trends, the big toe is playing an ever more starring role in foot balance, while the littlest toe is on its way out. We lean our weight on the big toe and expect it to do most of the work when we walk. It's only when it's out of commission that we feel compassion for it as we limp along. Abuse of the all-important big toe can create a common and unsightly problem: the bunion. With a bunion, the big toe leans toward the others rather than growing straight outward, and the deformed metatarsal joint then causes the bursal sac to become swollen and protrude.

When a bunion forms on the outside of the foot, by the little toe, it is known as a "bunionette," or "tailor's bunion"; the nickname derives from the erstwhile prevalence of these growths on the feet of cross-legged tailors. In general, the bunionette occurs together with the bunion as a sign of general foot imbalance.

Shoes emerge as the major villains here, especially the pointy, high-heeled variety that thrust the foot forward and exert enormous pressure upon the big toe. Studies reveal that barefooted peoples are less apt to develop bunions. So pressure on the big toe joint seems to be the definitive factor where bunions are concerned.

However, there is also a congenital condition which manifests itself as hypermobility of the forefoot. Instead of remaining in a fixed position, the big toe is able to bend at an extreme angle—in this case, growing sideways and not forward. The foot is then left open to the distortion of the first metatarsal bone. Children's feet should be checked for this predisposition; prevention is possible through the use of foot supports. As with most foot disorders, the basis of bunions is a biomechanical imbalance due to weak musculature, aggravated by a congenital factor or the vagaries of fashion.

The bunion not only looks unnatural—it usually feels that way. The surrounding tissue may ache, the second or third toe may hurt, and compensatory calluses due to incorrect bone alignment may form. The joint at the bunion's site may not hurt at all. If you are lucky, the only pain you feel will be the headache of adjusting your shoes to match the ever-changing map of your feet. In its chronic state, there is always the possibility of an acute pain attack. A bunion that "acts up" is simply letting you know that the bursal sac is inflamed.

Without surgery, the bunion will not go away. But is surgery the best option? That decision is up to you and your doctor, and as the list of options grows, your decision may be easier to make.

The tendency in modern medicine is to eliminate the problem permanently. However, since the foot takes longer to heal because of its low placement on the skeleton and its consequent unreliable circulation, most podiatrists tend to favor a conservative approach to start. Operating on your shoe may be easier than similar work on the foot; at least, it is not irreversible. As Hippocrates wrote: "Do as little as possible for maximum results." Removing the bunion surgically may not always be the best course of action since other factors (wide forefoot, bad circulation, etc.) must be taken into consideration and may not bode well.

In order to improve foot balance, different devices, such as toe jackets or toe sleeves, might alter the weight-bearing patterns of your feet. Latex shields that you can slip on your feet are also recommended to protect bunions from rubbing against shoes. Your doctor will make them to measure and they should last from one to two years. They are easily removed when you want to wash your feet since there is no paste involved as with over-the-counter type shields. Sometimes, when there is minimal discomfort, this device may prove entirely satisfactory. Unfortunately, only a relatively small number of bunion sufferers find relief from such shields; cortisone shots and hot water footbaths may be more to the point for more serious cases.

The type of bunion surgery you decide upon will depend on how you use your feet. If you have poor circulation, you can rule out surgery as a possibility since complete recovery would be too risky. If you are an avid athlete or ballerina, you will be more interested in correct bone alignment and proper foot function. But if you are simply concerned with improving your walking pattern, the process may be unexpectedly simple.

The most impressive advance in modern podiatry is the minimal incision ambulatory surgery, mentioned before. The success of this procedure depends largely upon the surgeon's expertise, since the bony enlargement itself is never actually seen. Working through a tiny hole, the surgeon makes the adjustment. Making miniature incisions is an art in itself since they do not exceed a ½ inch and yet they allow the surgeon to work on the basis of feel. Great care must be taken not to disturb the vein underneath the bunion. X-rays following surgery indicate excellent results in the majority of cases.

Using the same type of hypodermic as a dentist, the podiatrist numbs the bunion area with a fast-acting local anesthetic; nitrous oxide can be administered orally instead if the patient requests it. Special burs, also similar to dental tools, are used to grind away the protruding first metatarsal. The bur is inserted under the tissue of the small incision. Since the hole is so small, surrounding soft tissues and nerves are less traumatized. No stitches are needed; when the bandage is removed after a few days, the bunion will have been replaced by a small hole. Sometimes swelling may persist due to tissue swelling; don't mistake this for the bunion. It should disappear after a few months—although the wound may heal within days, bone takes months to catch up. Any discomfort can be easily soothed by taking simple aspirin. Once the scab falls off and the swelling subsides, street shoes can be worn again. Physiotherapy is then usually prescribed to speed recovery and improve circulation, although it is not absolutely necessary. Normal activity can be resumed at this point. Only one out of fifty bunion problems will recur according to recent statistics on the procedure. And best of all, no hospitalization is required. The entire operation takes place in the doctor's office and you can walk out afterward. Four days later the patient returns for a redressing.

The catch to the minimal incision procedure is that it *only* applies to *minimal* procedures: it can alleviate discomfort, but it does not repair toe function. It is not a replacement for the standard bunionectomy performed in a hospital, in which case the operation corrects the position of the first metatarsal. Office surgery is an outgrowth of an attempt to put podiatry on an equal footing with other branches of medicine. Because of the competitive atmosphere, specialists tend to snub podiatry; as a result, podiatrists found themselves upstaged by orthopedists—who are concerned with the entire human skeleton—for hospital space and turned to office work. Their results, although not as elaborate as certain hospital techniques, represent a large step for podiatry, as new procedures are instituted and made available to a wider range of patients.

A bunionectomy requires the correction of muscle and tendon alignment as well as that of the big toe metatarsal joint; total foot reconstruction is a much more ambitious procedure and takes much longer to heal. Soluble sutures eliminate the problem of getting stitches removed and the extent of scar tissue depends upon the surgeon's skill.

Some doctors believe that a fundamental principle of surgery is to be able to see what you are cutting. The type of procedure you decide upon depends largely on your podiatrist's stand on this matter. In a standard bunionectomy, hospital staff and services would be required and a complete physical exam would be needed; often unrelated problems are unearthed and complications sidestepped. Hospital stay can be minimized at an out-patient clinic: check-in usually starts at 7 A.M., which means release by noon. Medical insurance often covers most of the costs, whether you decide on a hospital or office procedure.

The key to your choice of surgery is the function of your foot in the future. If you feel that modifications on your shoes—such as cutting a hole in the toe box—are not giving you the mobility necessary to meet your daily needs, foot surgery may be the right step to take.

## RIGID TOE

Good toe movement means good cartilage. Once the cartilage between the toe joints begins to erode, repositioning the toe—which bunion surgery does—is not enough. The bone-on-bone contact needs cushioning.

The rigid toe, or hallux rigidus, requires this type of treatment. Either due to injury or obesity or common flatfeet, the big toe sometimes fuses with the metatarsal bone and creates an unnatural stiffness. Walking becomes a problem since the big toe has lost its flexibility. Perhaps a severe bunion is the underlying culprit or the bad habit of jamming the toe against the top of the shoe has engendered this condition. As the range of motion decreases, damage mounts. Attaching a metatarsal rocker bar to the bottom of the sole may ease walking, but a more permanent measure may mean greater comfort.

Joint replacement may be the answer. In order to release the locked joint, celastic (a silicone implant replacement) or polyethylene is inserted between the joints to reinstate movement. The process is simple and restores the function of the toe's bending motion. Without this flexibility, we would not be able to "toe off," the process of shifting all our weight onto the big toe in walking, which would severely limit our movements.

## Corns

"Since time immemorial the corn has created more wrinkles on the face than any other physical discomfort," declares Dr. Murray Weisenfeld, who has examined thousands of feet during his long career, including those of some pretty famous hoofers. "When it comes to a major foot complaint, the corn wins." In 1972 the National Center for Health Statistics put corns and calluses at the top of the list of prevalent disorders of the musculoskeletal system.

That the corn has been elevated to number one among foot ailments is no surprise; the love-hate relationship between the foot and the shoe has certainly helped the corn to attain its worldwide status. As John Gay wrote in 1716, "And when too short the modish shoes are worn, / You'll judge the seasons by your shooting corn." In ancient India, where the castor bean first grew, Brahmin physicians rubbed castor oil on their corns. To their great joy, the oil relieved soreness while keeping the tissue soft. Australian sheepherders preferred dandelion juice to cure their corns, while the Bavarians applied yeast of beer on their corns everyday for several weeks. Russians traditionally soaked black bread in vinegar and bound it to their corns for quick relief.

Corns appear in people of all ages, generally on the big or little toes where the shoe is more apt to make contact. Because of recurrent friction caused by the ill-fitting shoe, the irritated area receives an increase in blood supply which accelerates cell growth. Since the rubbing is centralized, the corn develops as a protective measure. The central "eye" of the irritation descends into the tissue in a conelike shape. The deeper the corn gets, the greater the possibility that it will poke a nerve if there is any external pressure on it. There is no "root" to the corn—this is simply an optical illusion generated by the central eye.

On the sunnier side, a corn will help forecast the weather. When the eye presses against a toe joint, bursitis may develop. This means that the bursa—the liquid-filled sac which protects the joint—is inflamed. If the atmospheric pressure decreases, as before a rainstorm, the already swollen bursa will expand even more

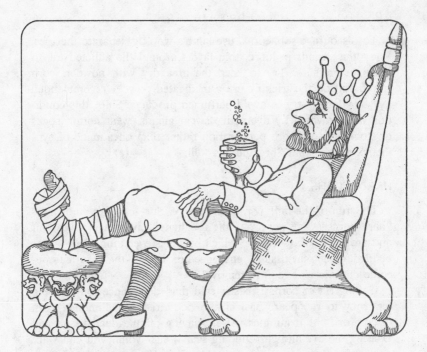

which will make you a walking weatherman—if a bit more uncomfortable.

Although shoes aggravate them, corns, like many other foot problems, are often symptomatic of other foot malfunctions. When the feet are out of line with the body, this imbalance may incorrectly distribute weight pressure onto the feet. Bad posture is the giveaway of faulty biomechanics and should be righted.

## SOFT CORNS

Frequently soft corns appear between the fourth and fifth toes as the result of pressure; one toe irritates its neighbor on a bony site and a corn erupts. In many cases, this type of corn occurs in pairs, one facing the other on neighboring toes. Or arthritis may enlarge the joints and encourage soft corns to develop. Since there is a tendency for body moisture to get caught between the toes, these corns feel rubbery and soft.

To discourage soft corns, use lamb's wool to separate the toes. Wrap the strands in loose, thin layers around the afflicted toe to alleviate pressure. Try to keep the area dry with powder; corn starch will do the trick or use a medicated powder recommended by your doctor—try to avoid perfumed products. Since this condition is aggravated by overactive sweat glands, wear cotton socks or stockings to absorb perspiration rather than ones made of synthetics which don't "breathe" as well.

## HARD CORNS

The run-of-the-mill corns on top of our toes are known as "hard corns." As they grow, the toughened outer layers wear off and are replaced by the eye which becomes ever more deeply embedded. Once scar tissue is ensconced in the toe, the corn may become chronic and require removal.

Getting rid of corns is easier said than done since they have a tendency to reappear. Basically, a podiatrist can eliminate corn discomfort within minutes. After shaving off the dead tissue and excising the eye and surrounding scar tissue—voilà! you can walk again. If a corn is particularly stubborn, it may mean joint surgery in order to return flexibility to the toe. Special power tools have been devised for this type of operation which requires an incision of about ½ inch and will leave only a small pinhole once healed.

If you have a very trustworthy pedicurist, he or she can perform a modified version of this procedure by shaving the corn down; but you must be absolutely sure that there is no underlying problem such as a tricky calcium deposit to complicate the procedure. If you choose to take matters into your own hands, results may take a different turn.

Bathroom techniques prove successful occasionally, but secondary problems occur more often. Doctors shudder at the thought of amateur surgery, but if you choose this method, be extremely cautious. Apply lanolin to soften the corn and make it less responsive to pressure. Read the ingredients list on the packaging of over-the-counter medications—if you have poor circulation, for example, acid corn plasters may incur secondary infections. Use corn pads carefully: the oval opening will force the corn to bulge into the hole and displace pressure in the area. A horseshoe-shaped pad behind the corn will be more effective since it protects against external pressure without creating new pressure. Cut your own pads from moleskin or foam rubber if you feel ambitious. Even a simple round adhesive pad may prove workable, if you place the pad over the corn. At night and while bathing, remove any covering to allow the tissue to breathe.

If you are a frustrated surgeon, the following procedure may prove a challenge to your skills; but if your instinct isn't on target, you may be in for a costly ride when complications set in after an unsuccessful operation. Prepare the area by applying a salicylic acid solution or similar caustic agent, then soak the foot in hot water for about fifteen minutes. Gently apply a pumice stone or emery board to the corn and work off the dead skin. Rasps and razors are definitely no-nos: corn "surgery" should be bloodless. Watch out not to damage underlying healthy tissue. Wash the foot again and blot dry. Repeat this procedure once or twice a week until the corn is visibly reduced and loosened enough to dislodge itself. If you detect any redness around the corn, discontinue use of the caustic until the normal pigment returns. Since you are not using the most sterile of facilities, this method may backfire—ulcerations may develop. So be good to yourself, and if the corn looks too advanced, visit a doctor.

Corns are not a fact of life—as long as you can account for the underlying reason, help is possible. If you find yourself buying larger and larger shoes to accommodate the corn, something is definitely amiss. The foot stops growing by age twenty or twenty-one. Roomier shoes may offer temporary appeasement, but eliminating the cause will be more efficient. Adjust the biomechanical problems and leave this problem behind.

## Calluses

Like a corn, a callus, or tyloma, develops to protect the foot against the elements (external friction and pressure), only this time on a diffuse area. Think of it as a chronic blister. Without pressure, a callus could not exist. If you are bedridden for a prolonged time, you will notice how calluses abate. Whereas a corn is cone-shaped, a callus grows on flat surfaces and has no nucleus. Most often, a callus appears on the weight-bearing parts of the foot, such as the heel or ball, or beneath the joints.

Not everyone has calluses on their feet. Long periods of standing may contribute to their development, as well as participating in sports which may require unwieldy footwear such as ski boots. Naturally, a person who pads about barefoot on rough surfaces is more likely to have protective callus growth on the sole than the average shoe wearer. When a callus appears on the shod foot, this is a sign of incorrect weight distribution. The age-old villain high-heeled shoes tilt the foot at a very precarious angle, causing the ball of the foot to smooth over into a large callus. Rather than being distributed evenly through the foot, most of the body's weight lands on the metatarsal area—just asking for complications.

As long as the callus is not painful, the foot imbalance is nothing to worry about—at least, for the moment. Basically, any callus formation indicates some degree of imbalance: weak ankles may cause the heel to rotate and develop a large callus for stability, or a foot that leans inward may have a large callus along the side of the big toe. A red, swollen rim around the callus will alert the foot owner to any unhappy developments. Even "chauffeur's callus," which builds up from long hours working car brakes and, in some models, clutch pedals, may ache and require professional treatment. Redness indicates inflammation, which increases the amount of blood in that area, easily caused by the friction between a hard surface and the foot.

When there is a burning sensation in the callus, congestion and swelling under it is irritating the nerve endings. (The callus itself cannot burn since it consists only of dead cells.) This unpleasant symptom may be a warning of anemia, poor circulation, diabetes, or a vitamin deficiency. Sometimes the burning sensation is due to a corn growing within the callus, especially on the ball of the foot. In this case, often localized pressure has been added to general pressure and may displace a metatarsal bone. For relief, attach a metatarsal pad to the area.

Although pedicures are relaxing and help to keep calluses at a minimum, severe calluses can only be helped by eliminating their cause. The remedy may be quite simple. For example, one leg may be a fraction shorter than the other and may compensate by developing heavier calluses. A shoe support or insole will soon alleviate this imbalance.

If surgery is required in chronic, deep-seated cases, the doctor will use one of two approaches: either cutting off the callus in one segment by loosening it from the healthy layer of skin and chiseling it away; or, more often, chiseling it off in small slices.

## Fallen Arches

Standing is no fun. We do it all the time: in stores, on buses, in crowds. Our feet are obliged to keep our bulk upright without relief; and sometimes we expect them to carry an inordinate amount of weight, too. The ligaments, tough fibroelastic tissues responsible for holding the foot in one piece, soon weaken. Improper shoes also contribute to this fatigue. As the ligaments give way, the longitudinal heel-to-toe arch lowers with them; stress also registers in the lower back and a swayback may develop. In fact, back pain is a very common sign of this type of foot trouble.

You can check your longitudinal arch by examining the relationship of your knee to your ankle and foot. If the midpoints do not form a more or less straight line, you have an arch problem. The foot may be turning outward until your body weight is resting on the longitudinal arch instead of on the toes and heel. The foot should work like a tripod, supporting body weight on the heel, the first toe and the last toe.

If you suffer from foot pain during the day or your soles seem to "burn," strain is taking its toll on your longitudinal arches and they are about to give way.

To build up strength in your longitudinal arches, do simple exercises. Try toe curling and stretching; foot rotation will help, too. Orthotics or commercial arch supports may also provide extra support to sagging ligaments. If the condition is in the earlier stages, clogs may be able to help by supplying a rigid platform for the sole. Wooden exercise sandals may also help to give the muscles a workout. Maurita Robarge, a Dr. Scholl's foot-comfort appliance consultant, additionally suggests shaking out each foot vigorously for one minute a day to relax the muscles and then pausing before flexing the toes and exercising the muscles and ligaments.

## Hammertoes

A hammertoe looks like a little hammer in a piano: the medial joints bend so that the toe rises above the other toes and the top joint is almost curled under. The tendons and ligaments contract to such an extent that they pull the front of the toe backward. This affliction seems most common in the second toe. There is a congenital element here which manifests itself as a biomechanical disorder—high-arched feet are more inclined to develop hammertoes because of the positioning of the ligaments.

And shoes are no help. Except for the big toe, the other toes are an open target for shoe pressure. Sometimes narrow, pointed shoes compress a latent hammertoe into existence by forcing ligaments into unnatural positions. Such constriction may even cause foot muscles to waste away by depriving them of movement.

If a tendency for hammertoes is recognized in your foot, its natural flexibility allows correction by the application of simple pressure—with a splint or similar device. Exercises to lengthen the foot tendons and stretch the Achilles tendon area will help fight hammertoes as well.

With age, a hammertoe becomes more and more rigid and surgery may be required to correct it. The podiatrist can perform an arthroplasty to straighten the toe by removing a wedge of bone from the angle in which the toe is unnaturally held; or the doctor may opt for lengthening the tendons. A minimal incision operation is simple and painless, giving the hammertoe owner an alternative to living in misery. Discomfort may occur during the healing process if there is swelling, but proper medications keep pain in check. And when the ultimate result is pain-free walking, who can complain?

## Heels

The heel takes the brunt of our unsteady walking habits. Although it is the largest bone in the foot, the heel bone is still smaller than a golf ball. Between the bone and the sole lies ⅜ inch of soft protective tissue which is easily worn down. The running foot especially tends to try the heel; by exerting three times your weight on your heel, the effect is comparable to the pounding of a sledgehammer against an unyielding surface—in this case often the pavement. Walking also takes its toll on the heel bone since leg muscles connecting it to the Achilles tendon may become strained.

### "PUMP BUMP"

Most commonly, bony growths develop on the heel bone because of the foot's archenemy: tight shoes. If the heel thrusts outward to an exaggerated degree, resultant friction will cause a "pump bump," or bony protrusion. Unrestricted motion of the heel will have the same effect. This bump generally appears at the point where the Achilles tendon connects with the heel. There should be no pain—until the bump gets inflamed. Pain is then proportionate to the size of the growth and the intensity of the inflammation. Treatment consists mainly of protecting the heel from further rubbing against the shoe by wearing a larger size shoe equipped with a heel lift to stabilize the foot and accommodate the bump. Your doctor may recommend cortisone shots to relieve symptoms but they will not cure the problem.

### HEEL SPURS

A heel spur is also a bony growth caused by a biomechanical disorder; but it is distinguished from the pump bump by its position on the underside of the heel bone. Spurs are thought to be the logical result of a torn longitudinal ligament which bleeds and generates fibrous tissue that ultimately calcifies. If the foot lists too far in one direction, for example, the strain on its muscles may tear ligaments which then bleed and calcify into a bony protrusion. Overweight people tend to develop spurs, probably because of excess weight bearing down on their heels.

Occasionally, spurs appear without warning. The accompanying pain is equally mysterious; generally, pain strikes when the foot is in action and the injured ligament is forced to stretch. The muscles near the heel bone then get inflamed and add to general distress. To ease the pain, insert a small pad cut from a piece of foam rubber under your heel when you wear shoes. This little pad should be designed with a small depression in the center to accommodate the spur.

If inflammation is severe, your doctor may recommend an immediate cortisone injection to provide quick relief. He or she can then strap your foot to correct the imbalance; or you can opt for shoe supports. As the very last resort, surgery is possible. But since heel spurs are not potentially dangerous, only crippling pain should prompt this course of action. The best thing you can do is to rest and elevate your foot, allowing the muscles to relax. A hot compress would be soothing since the blood vessels would then dilate and circulation would be stimulated.

Inflammation of the longitudinal arch, or plantar fasciitis, might precede the appearance of a heel spur, since stress may cause the plantar fascia, the fibrous tissue fanning from the heel to the toes, to become inflamed. Again, rest is the most expedient course of action; strapping and ultrasound techniques may help as well. The ultrasound method works by spraying sound waves at a very high frequency on the afflicted area; in this way, deep body tissues can be "massaged" and pain may be reduced. Time is the most important element in the healing of spurs; be patient and rest your heels when you can to allow the spur time to abate.

## PAINFUL FEET

As women approach menopause, their bodies undergo many changes. Often, a syndrome resulting in painful feet occurs: fissures appear on the heels and, depending upon the degree of severity, will crack or even bleed. Short, overweight body types seem prone to have this problem, perhaps since their feet are over-worked by excess baggage.

Hormonal changes may also contribute to this phenomenon, but as yet there are no known medical reasons for it. The best immediate course of action for the sufferer would be to apply a lubricant to her feet nightly and then wrap them in plastic to soften hardened skin. Vegetable shortening, hand cream, or salicylic acid preparations may work to heal the area. After a week of this procedure, apply petroleum jelly instead, again keeping the feet wrapped to ensure better absorption during the night. Within two weeks, if the condition does not visibly improve consult your doctor.

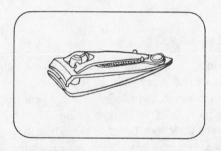

## Toenails

Toenails have a rough time. Unlike fingernails—which we tend to pamper—we tend to hide toenails inside our shoes without a second thought to their appearance. They are subjected to stubbing, falling objects, and visiting fungi. When hangnails appear (those nasty slivers of dead skin on the borders of our nails), we may tug them off thoughtlessly, asking for an inflammation, rather than taking the time to trim them off neatly. White marks under the toenails come and go, attesting to recurrent injuries or nutritional deficiencies. We usually ignore them completely. If the nail on the big toe hits the top of the shoe repeatedly, it may thicken (and become a "club nail." As long as we don't have to see our toenails chipping away and turning strange colors, we may think we don't have to take the responsibility for their well-being.

Problems with toenails cannot be traced to genetic factors or even that old standby, tight shoes. It's simply a matter of good hygiene. And once you abuse a toenail, no amount of bathroom surgery is going to restore it to health.

The nail emerges from the matrix, an area beneath the skin that is not visible, and grows up over the nail bed—the skin which shows through the transparent part of the nail. Nails grow slowly; weeks may pass before they advance ¼ inch. Once the nail grows past the nail bed, it appears as the white edge. Depending upon how we treat this edge, the nail's appearance will be attractive or not.

## INGROWN TOENAILS

Most commonly, once people decide to deal with their toenails, they tend to get carried away with the nail clipper. Doctors regard teenagers and men as most apt to be avid clippers who don't consider the consequences of careless clipping. These become painfully obvious once their toes begin to throb. Keep in mind that if you snip in haste, you may have to repent at leisure. The big toenail is the victim in the majority of cases, being subject to more shoe pressure than the other toes—although by no means does it have exclusive rights.

The correct way to cut a toenail is simply straight across, with the outer edge parallel to the top of the toe. Do not cut the nail shorter than the end of the toe and always smooth the edge with an emery board. Trimming the toenail too close to the quick and rounding the corners will often produce an ingrown toenail. Convex nails are more vulnerable than flat ones since they can be more easily irritated by external pressure. Socks and support hose can aggravate ingrown toenails, too. Whenever the toes are cramped together, the flesh around the nails will press against them, making it seem as if the nail is growing out of the flesh. Actually, the nail is breaking into the skin—and that hurts!

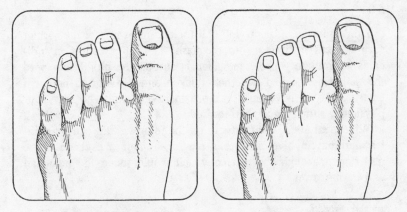

Battered toenails.                    Proper pedicure.

As long as infection is not present, you can separate the nail from the impinging skin by inserting several strands of absorbent cotton between them. To put the cotton in place, use the blunt end of an orange stick. By relieving the pressure this way, you can sidestep more serious conditions. The application of an antibacterial or antifungal agent, such as gentian violet solution, may prevent infection. Sometimes a callus forms as nature's own protective measure. If this happens, insert a small piece of cotton beneath the nail to encourage nail growth. Do not remove the callus. If you do, you remove a natural shield and may risk infection.

If a raw, red area develops around the ingrown nail, pus may be present and you will then be dealing with a full-fledged infection. For immediate relief, soak the foot in warm—not hot—water three times a day if possible, for ten minutes each time. Your foot will rightly resist tight shoes during this siege, so wear an open sandal if you can. The sooner you hobble to the podiatrist, the easier you will make it for your foot. Fooling around with home cures will probably complicate the infection. If you try to trim the offending part of the nail yourself, spicules of nail may irritate the nail groove further and "proud flesh"—painful tissue—will result. Cutting a V-shape from the center of the nail in accordance with the old wives' tale will not encourage the nail to grow inward, thus drawing it away from the raw area; in fact, it will do no good whatsoever.

Don't mistake an incurving nail for an ingrown one; the former seems to curve directly into the flesh. The latter condition indicates a circulatory problem which is cutting the blood supply to the nail bed; the bed will then thicken and a distorted nail will emerge. If you have one or more incurving nails, consult your physician; surgery may be required.

With local anesthesia, surgery on the ingrown nail can be painless and may involve excision of part of the nail or excision of the nail down through the matrix—which would mean the new nail will be narrower.

INFECTED NAILS

The two main causes of toenail infection are bacteria and fungi. Paronychia is a bacterial condition due to such nasty invaders as streptococci or staphylococci. It appears as a pimple on the cuticle and many simply remain in this dormant pale red stage. As long as you leave the pimple alone, it will leave you alone. Once it is irritated, the best thing to do is soak the nail in hot water and treat the infection as a pimple by gently allowing pus to drain. Be careful since the types of bacteria causing paronychia are notorious for causing blood poisoning.

If you have chronic paronychia, avoid damp conditions and friction on the infected nails. A 1 to 2 per cent gentian violet solution in alcohol applied several times a day may be recommended by your podiatrist to relieve discomfort.

Onychomycosis, a fungal condition, is ringworm of the nail plate. It was considered incurable until recently when it was found to respond to medications designed for the skin. Usually it occurs in a toenail concurrently with athlete's foot, another fungal disease, although the two complaints may make solo appearances since dormant fungi can act up at different times. Skin diseases such as psoriasis often infect the nails, although nail infections may take a much longer time to clear up.

Incipient signs of onychomycosis include a change in the color of the toenail to a lusterless, chalky, or yellowish shade, and a distinct odor. As the fungus spreads, it may infect the entire nail until the nail edge looks granular and acquires a sandlike texture. Soon the nail seems to rise from the nail bed and then you are forced to deal with it. If it spreads to all your nails—fingernails as well as toenails—you will have your hands full. If you ignore it, the infection may decide to move to other fungus-loving places, such as the groin, by hitching a ride under a fingernail. Then you will have what is known as a "mixed" infection.

The first step back to health is to treat the toenails. You can coat the nail edge with an antifungal agent, but it is advisable to leave this procedure in the hands of a qualified podiatrist. The chances of success are greater if an expert is in charge. However, no topically applied agent seems thoroughly reliable and doctors are still testing for the best one.

## SPLITTING NAILS

Nemesis to many a stocking, the split toenail is a nuisance. In this case, overcleanliness may be responsible. By bathing your feet every day, your toenails may alternately soften and harden to an extreme. This can cause the nails to become brittle and crack. Damp conditions may aggravate the condition.

Of course, there is no pat solution to this annoying problem, except to avoid soaking your feet once they've been washed. Your podiatrist may prescribe an ointment to prevent the nails from hardening. Contrary to popular belief, gelatin has no remedial effect on the nails; in fact, it has no significant effect at all. Its protein content may promote nail growth, but so will any protein-packed food; as long as you're getting the right daily amount, there should be no reason for a supplement. So consider Jell-O a dessert, not a nail cure. Above all, do not pull at or pick your nails. Many people tend to pull off split nails, especially when they are somewhat loose. This habit may come back to haunt you in your sleep.

# RUBBING THE WRONG WAY
## Skin Diseases

## Athlete's Foot

If persistent blisters with oozing fluid are dogging your steps, the three possible causes are: fungal infections, allergies, or eczema. Most often it is the fungal infection athlete's foot, the most common skin malady in the United States. It can be easily identified by checking its favorite hangout between the fourth and fifth toes: after irritating that area, the fungus usually spreads to the sole of the foot. Since it is contagious, it is likely to affect both feet. In this way, you can sometimes distinguish it from an allergy. If only one foot is bothering you, you probably have an allergic reaction, which requires different medical attention from that of athlete's foot. Athletes are not the only ones vulnerable to this condition; in fact, the name was the brainchild of several clever ad men who wanted to glamorize an otherwise unsightly problem. Bad circulation, obesity, arthritis, and diabetes may all contribute to its appearance. If you wear closed, leather shoes all year round, athlete's foot may be a hazard.

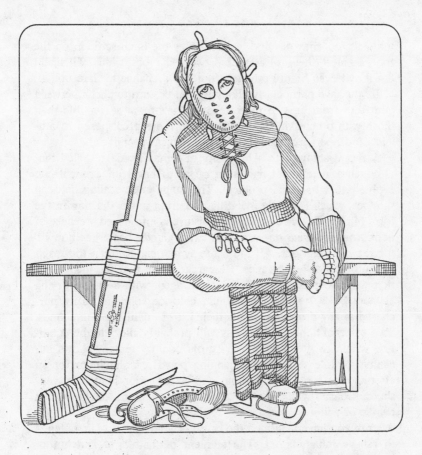

There are twenty species of fungi which may be responsible for athlete's foot. Treatment varies with the type and number of fungi present. Since the condition is communicable and known to lurk about public showers in wait for the unsuspecting bare sole, wear some kind of foot covering if you patronize them.

If you contract athlete's foot, between the peeling and scratching, your feet assume a focal position in your life—much to your dismay. Once the blisters explode, the skin becomes crusty and even less appetizing. An acute attack is typified by a sudden itching, burning, or "prickly" sensation. The skin becomes scaly and cracks and the condition is only aggravated by scratching. Chronic athlete's foot may develop insidiously as the fungi settle in on the foot. Be alert, then, for a crack between the toes, which will signal the threat even before athlete's foot has a chance to flare up.

If you have particularly alkaline skin, be sure to check between your toes from time to time since you are more susceptible than those with other skin types. Men seem more predisposed to athlete's foot, perhaps because of this chemical peculiarity.

A recent study at the University of Pennsylvania revealed that although athlete's foot may start off as a fungal infection, it can evolve into a bacterial problem. The fungi cause scaling between the toes, which is mildly irritating and erupt under the skin in the form of blisters. Once excessive moisture is introduced, because of nonporous footwear or overactive sweat glands, bacteria elbow in, forcing the fungi out. All the acute symptoms are then the result of the bacterial interference. Researchers feel that the ideal solution would consist of an antibacterial agent with a strong drying element. A 30 per cent aluminum chloride solution, easily purchased at any drugstore, heads their list of qualifying compounds. Two external applications a day will probably alleviate the condition within two to three days. An old country remedy shows uncanny good sense by recommending powdered aluminum for an after-shower foot-dusting ritual and as an odor fighter in your shoes. Consult your doctor for recommendations on your best course of action.

Until you have identified the cause of your rash, the first step is to relieve inflammation. The eminent dermatologist and author Dr. Jonathan Zizmor recommends a simple method: Fill a quart bottle with a 90 per cent ice and 10 per cent milk mixture. Add two teaspoons of salt and stir. Apply a compress soaked in this to the raw area, using a clean, white cotton cloth, until itching abates. After the discomfort subsides, apply zinc ointment. And be good to your feet; keep them uncovered and try to rest them so as not to disturb the tissue any further. Elevating your feet will also help reduce any swelling. Working with the assumption that the fungus is still present, you can apply preparations which contain an effective antifungal chemical such as tolnaftate.

The U. S. Army has experimented for years to find an efficacious medication to win the infantryman's endless struggle against athlete's foot. Before tolnaftate became widely available, undecylenic acid was recruited to do the job. A 1971 AMA report stated that there are more than a hundred over-the-counter preparations for fungus infections, but consult your doctor before you buy and be an educated consumer before you decide to treat your foot ailments. The old-fashioned method was to rely on salicylic acid to peel off the infection, but when it comes to foot comfort, it pays to be up-to-date and use the newer, perhaps more effective products.

To prevent athlete's foot, keep your feet dry and try to alternate footwear. Clean between your toes and use a powder on your feet and in your shoes. Shepherds are said to place lamb's wool between their toes to absorb moisture, dampening the wool with grated garlic or garlic juices, as a natural antibiotic. The key to foot health here is cleanliness; the method you choose is up to you.

## Allergies

Allergic reactions in the foot arise for myriad reasons. One mysterious syndrome was recently traced to a poison sumac used by East Indians to tan buffalo-hide sandals which were then sold on the American market, causing an unusual epidemic. More often dyes used in socks and shoes—Bismarck brown in particular —or synthetic materials are responsible; nail polish and foot deodorants may also irritate. Although allergic symptoms can resemble those found with athlete's foot, it is important to distinguish allergy from fungus since treatment will be different. Generally, the circumstances are predictable: the foot perspires heavily and because of friction with the shoe, absorbs unfriendly chemicals. If you suffer from a foot allergy, consider all factors: Have you bought a new pair of shoes lately? Do your feet only itch when you wear a certain pair? Or is it your socks?

Usually in an allergic reaction the offensive material tends to leave a well-defined impression on the foot. Frequently it leaves its mark on the tops of the toes or the midfoot, where the foot has had direct contact with the shoe. Uncallused areas are particularly vulnerable to allergies. Slowly, red patches will develop, bumps may soon follow, and finally itchiness or blisters will appear.

The majority of allergies can be attributed to chemicals used in shoe manufacturing. Most common is the rubber toe-box syndrome. Rubber is mainly used in the toe box and in adhesives fastening the inner sole. Nickel reinforcements in the toe box may also irritate the foot. A dermatologist can give you a patch test for nickel, or you can simply wear a piece of nickel jewelry to test your reaction. Heel stiffeners may also disturb sensitive skin. Tanning agents containing formaldehyde or chromates are also allergenic. An estimated 8 per cent of the United States population is allergic to potassium dichromate, a common ingredient in tanned leather.

Chronic allergy cases may simply manifest themselves in mild redness while the offensive material is present. An acute allergic attack is usually accompanied by burning and swelling. The skin will crack and peel unless the allergy is properly dealt with, possibly resulting in a secondary infection if you're not careful.

Your susceptible foot should be kept as dry as possible. This may mean wearing two layers of hosiery; the air spaces between them will absorb sweat more efficiently while padding the foot more securely. Avoid synthetic hosiery when possible. After your physician has identified the cause of your allergy—either with a standardized shoe-chemical patch test or by the process of elimination of the obvious possibilities—your only recourse is to expel the offending material from your wardrobe. A congenial foot environment must be maintained at all times. Use very mild soaps, preferably the nonallergenic type.

If you have an ultrasensitive foot, special shoes that do not contain any of the offensive chemicals or materials that may cause an allergic outbreak may be the answer. Sources of such shoes around the country include:

Prescription Footwear Association, P. O. Box 54696, Atlanta, Ga. 30308

Julius Altschul, Inc., 117 Gratten St., Brooklyn, N.Y. 11237

Alden Shoe Company, Taunton St., Middleboro, Mass. 02346

Foot-So-Port Company, Oconomowoc, Wis. 53066

## Eczema — Dry Skin

Although eczema must be treated by a doctor, you can learn how to treat certain types of dry skin yourself. Itchy, dry skin on your feet may develop after other conditions, especially the fungal variety, clear up. A podiatrist from San Francisco, Dr. Donald Nash, has experimented with urea and discovered that in certain forms it may provide relief in such cases. By stimulating the water uptake of the skin, it promotes peeling of toughened skin. Urea preparations are obtainable over-the-counter and should alleviate the annoying problem of dry, flaky skin if used regularly. Petroleum jelly preparations are also effective as immediate measures.

## Warts

Warts are benign tumors generated by viruses; the specific culprits have not yet been apprehended. Warts appear as rubbery-looking corns with uneven textures. There is a psychogenic factor which shows that warts are likely to appear during stressful times. This is one condition where mind over matter may work. In children especially, some "voodoo" panaceas seem to work. Early in the twentieth century suggestions were made that hypnosis could help to remove warts. The latter premise was shelved until recently when Massachusetts General Hospital conducted a controlled study with interesting results. The group being studied comprised seventeen patients with an average of thirty warts apiece. A control group of seven patients who did not undergo hypnosis were retained for observation. Once a week for five weeks the seventeen patients were hypnotized and losing their warts was suggested. Nine showed great improvement after this experiment, with loss of all warts in four cases. The smaller control group showed no change. But still there is no wide-reaching conclusive evidence that hypnosis is the answer—after all, not everyone is eager to undergo hypnosis even if it means living wart-free.

Warts seem to favor wet places. According to podiatrists, foot warts reach epidemic proportions in the autumn—a logical consequence of a barefoot summer season. The bathroom is an all-time favorite hiding place for wart-bearing viruses; dorm showers are also suspect.

Like corns, warts on the foot grow in a conic shape and prefer areas of abnormal pressure on the sole. Underfoot they tend to grow inward—unlike warts on other parts of the body—and thereby develop a spongy quality. They are called "plantar warts" in honor of the region they have invaded—the plantar surface of the foot, or the sole. (Most people have heard of this foot ailment, but mistake it for a farmer's woe.)

At first, a plantar wart may feel like a random pebble in your shoe. But it likes company, and the central wart often surrounds itself with satellites. On occasion, the group coalesces and gives a "mosaic" appearance, sometimes usurping most of the sole.

There is no one definitive way for the podiatrist to remove a plantar wart. In fact, there are at least a dozen choices. Most efficient is an electric needle that excises the wart and kills the offensive viruses—a crucial step as leftover viral material will cause the wart to recur. And there is no lengthy inconvenience such as the need to avoid getting the area wet. Bandages can be removed within a week and permanent correction should be established.

At the University of California in Los Angeles, Dr. J. H. Greenberg has been testing a chemical compound that would make the body's immune system ward off invasion by wart-generating viruses. This substance—DNCB—was tested on the warts of five patients, four of whom showed vast improvement.

Vitamin A acid has been proven very effective against flat warts, especially the stubborn sort. Tests at the University of Iowa show a 0.05 per cent solution of Vitamin A acid to work if applied twice a day. For tough plantar warts, glutaraldehyde in a 25 per cent solution will harden the wart to make shaving it down easier. Within three months, the problem should be licked. But until these methods are perfected, they are only available under a physician's jurisdiction.

Warts are curious entities with unpredictable response mechanisms. That's why home remedies abound, and there is no reason why they shouldn't work to some degree. Edgar Cayce, the legendary American healer, suggested daily applications of a paste made of baking soda mixed with castor oil. In the past, cures have included such far-out procedures as soaking the foot in urine or rubbing potato slices against the area.

In a more modern vein, if you enjoy home remedies for toe warts, start by protecting the wart with a small felt pad to relieve pressure from above while "coaxing" it out. In addition to the pad, wear a plaster—cut to size—containing a 20 to 40 per cent salicylic acid solution. Wear the plaster for twelve hours maximum, so as not to irritate the surrounding skin. Then soak your feet for ten to twenty minutes in warm water, gently working a pumice stone over the wart to remove dead skin. This process takes weeks, or even months, depending upon the size of the wart; but if you are careful and follow the routine religiously, success should be in the offing. However, home remedies are often not as efficacious as professional procedures. Consult your doctor before you attempt a cure.

If you decide to swim during treatment, Dr. Elizabeth Roberts suggests coating the wart with clear nail polish to keep it dry. Eventually the polish will peel off by itself, and that way, no harm will be done.

# INVISIBLE
# PROBLEMS
## What Goes On
## Inside

## Cold Feet

Although we all get cold feet from time to time, suffering them on a daily basis becomes a problem. From bed warmers to electric blankets man has learned to cope with icy feet. Usually we attribute them to bad circulation, which is true—in part. When there is no pain, however, the circulation is not fully to blame. Natural warmth derives from the blood flow originating in the deeper reaches of the body. Blood then circulates to the skin by means of capillaries from the small arteries through one's tissues. This movement is controlled by the sympathetic nervous system; if the system hinders the flow, the feet will cool. In some people the sympathetic nervous system is more unevenly active than in others and may inhibit the warming blood flow. Drinking coffee or smoking cigarettes can affect the nerves to the detriment of the feet (and hands) by distracting the blood flow. Nicotine and caffeine close blood vessels down and slow circulation; since the feet are

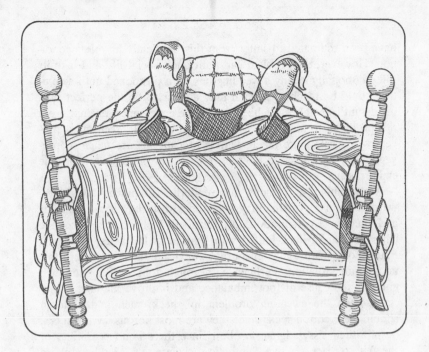

always the first to suffer at diminished blood flow, being low men on the totem pole, they soon grow cold.

Sometimes external factors contribute to our cold feet, as in the case of frostbite or chilblains. The best antidote here is to rub those frozen tootsies with boric acid or lanolin ointment; a hot soak will also serve to stimulate blood flow into the lower reaches.

Another type of cold foot is the one that perspires to excess and then cools off to an uncomfortable degree. This sweating—called hyperhidrosis—may simply indicate uncontrollable sweating all over the body. Triggered by the nerves, the sweat glands stimulate perspiration in the palms and soles, as well as in the armpits and groin. In some cases, the feet are the main target. Perhaps the handiest remedy is a foot deodorant much like the underarm sort, or use a powder in your shoes to counteract moisture.

A variation of this condition is bromidrosis, more widely known as "smelly feet." Perhaps unfairly, this problem has been nicknamed the "husband's disease"; roughly 80 million Americans have been estimated to suffer from this physically harmless condition. However, the problem can limit one's social life and take its toll emotionally. Many a wedding has been postponed until a solution could be reached. A man may appear to be the perfect husband—until he takes off his shoes. Nor are women exempt from this problem. Romance may be upstaged by smelly feet unless preventive measures are taken. Unless precautions are taken to prevent soggy skin between the toes, removal of one's shoes could be embarrassing.

Any number of reasons may underlie bromidrosis. Calluses, warts, or other growths may sometimes disturb walking patterns and encourage perspiration. Dr. Elizabeth Roberts recognizes the Charlie Chaplin duck-footed walk as one of the worst offenders. Faulty foot posture may encourage sweat glands and result in this unpleasant situation. Perhaps a thorough foot examination will uncover the cause of foot imbalance and improve matters.

To keep the sweating problem in check, men and children should wear cotton socks since they are most porous. White socks, despite their sissy stigma, are best since there is no possibility of the skin to react to a dye. Synthetic socks are out. Also helpful are foot soaks in a solution of cool water mixed with aluminum acetate. Podiatrists may administer zinc sulphate electrical baths to shrink the sweat glands and thereby reduce sweating.

If your feet are limiting your social life, new grooming techniques may be the solution. In addition to washing your feet well and drying them carefully on at least a daily basis, you might wear something in your shoes to prevent odor. A layer of soft latex blended with activated charcoal works to pick up offensive odors from the feet, shoes, and hosiery.

But the key to bromidrosis often is "Relax!"

## Cramps

How many times have you cried out in agony and hopped about yelping incoherently in response to the intense pain in your foot? This pain will probably recur from time to time. Suddenly your toes feel as if they are being stretched away from each other and then there you are again—dancing around in pain.

Dr. Bernard Rosenstein says that severe foot cramps provide a major impetus for many of his patients to visit him. Generally, the patient assumes that the problem lies in poor circulation. Actually it is unrelated to any disease. A cramp of this type is simply a muscle spasm due to fatigue and a certain kind of chemical build-up that results from improper walking habits. The excess work muscles must perform because of a lopsided gait, for example, causes chemicals to collect and irritate nerve endings; lactic acid is a main suspect here. (Lack of oxygen flow to the muscle will cause lactic acid to build up.) The spasm usually occurs shortly after a stretching movement or following a prolonged period of discomfort. Often, trying a new sport may strain a muscle which will then react in this manner. The afflicted foot is generally overworking to compensate for an imbalance. Gradually this problem intensifies and sometimes will occur on a nightly basis.

The fatigue spasm likes to creep up unannounced, when you least expect it—while you sleep, for example, or even when you are unwinding in an armchair. Suddenly your foot decides that it's had enough and it wants to let you know.

For quick relief, the best thing to do is to stand on a cold surface or wrap your foot in a cold towel. Massage will also soothe it. Oral doses of quinine sulfate are often prescribed by physicians for night cramps, but this treatment will only erase the symptom, not the cause. It would be more to the point to correct whatever is bothering your foot to begin with and enjoy activity without the threat of future cramps.

## INTERMITTENT CLAUDICATION

If you find that leg and foot cramps occur during activity, it may be a sign of atherosclerosis. Only your physician can determine this. In atherosclerosis the arteries in the feet and legs are blocked to the extent that the necessary amount of oxygen for the muscles cannot be sustained—not even while walking. Cramping or an achy feeling may force the walker to pause until enough oxygen reaches the lower extremities. In this way walking becomes a matter of stopping and starting at patterned intervals. Since the pain occurs only when movement is introduced, it is called "intermittent claudication"—or limping at timed intervals.

Once the condition worsens, it may become painful, even for the resting foot. Without the help of gravity, the blood may have a difficult time getting down into the feet; for this reason, it is important to walk whenever possible and massage the feet to encourage the blood to flow downward. The foot also becomes more vulnerable to infection and injury because the defense mechanisms are numbed by decreased circulation. Home cures may jeopardize the foot; hot soaks are the worst possible thing to try since they prevent oxygen from entering the oxygen-deprived foot.

Your physician may send you to a vascular specialist who can advise you as to the degree of blockage due to atherosclerosis and whether a bypass operation would be advisable. In less severe cases, the best course of action may be to pamper your feet by eliminating tight shoes and boots. Never elevate the legs since this will diminish the downward blood flow; support hose and garters are equally harmful to this condition.

For best results, your doctor will probably suggest that you follow these simple rules:

1   Twice a day, relax your feet in a tub of *warm* water; massage them underwater and clean with mild soap.

2   After the bath, swab the feet down with rubbing alcohol and complete the treatment with a coat of lanolin and some talc.

3  Try to keep your feet warm and avoid extremes in temperature.

4  Adopt a low-fat diet.

5  *Don't smoke under any circumstances.*

## Circulation Disorders

DIABETES

Gravity does its best to pull the blood to the feet when we are standing up but cannot ensure a roundtrip ticket: often there is a stasis of blood, which means that the flow slows down considerably. In the diabetic, the situation is further complicated by faulty sugar metabolization, making the blood circulation even more sluggish. Arteries in the foot harden and narrow prematurely, permanently damaging the peripheral nerves. The resultant loss of sensation makes injury an ever dangerous possibility.

Diabetes appears in middle-aged people (roughly ages forty to sixty) about ten times more often than among younger adults, and it most often strikes women. Victims usually manifest subtle symptoms of the disease at first and the condition of the feet may be an important clue in controlling it.

With age, the incidence of diabetes triples. A person over sixty is more prone to hardened arteries and poor blood circulation, which are both aggravated by the diabetic condition. The feet then become an easy target for infection.

Because of diminished nerve response, diabetics are more vulnerable to severe problems that may develop before any pain registers. And since the foot recovers more slowly than other parts of the body, this may mean serious complications, such as gangrene. Until skin and underlying tissues manifest signs of gangrene, the diabetic may notice nothing amiss. Initial signs of such a condition would include superficial ulcerations accompanied by scaly skin, dry nails or skin, and general numbness. The ulcerations (breaks in the tissue) allow further deterioration of deeper tissues to spread. Most often such ulcerations are found on the ball of the foot which is an easy target for unstable walking patterns. Or they can appear on a callused area. One of the first symptoms of diabetes is an ulceration that does not heal. Consult your physician since hospitalization may be required. The diabetic's skin has a tendency toward dryness which can be counteracted with a prescribed emollient or simple lanolin. But without proper medical attention, secondary infections may set in and inflammation can easily spread through the foot and leg. If infection is not treated at once, the problem may become one of life or death.

Toenails of diabetics are equally vulnerable. This is why most podiatrists recommend that diabetics have their toenails trimmed at a doctor's office to be safe. A monthly visit at the very least would be necessary to ensure a diabetic's foot health.

Statistics show that in at least 50 per cent of diabetic gangrene cases, tissue damage was avoidable. If you are a diabetic and adhere to these general rules, you can decrease the odds of contracting a crippling foot infection:

1   Wash your feet daily with soap and warm water; pat them dry and massage them with a lubricant.

2   If your toenails are brittle, soak and cream them but do not cut them yourself.

3   Never use corn or callus medications or any antiseptic that is not prescribed for you by your doctor.

4   Keep your feet warm: wear socks at night if necessary but avoid heat pads since a diabetic's perception of heat is often inaccurate.

5   Do not walk barefoot; inspect your feet daily for possible injury.

6   Only wear leather shoes; avoid shoes made of nonporous materials such as plastics, reptile skin, or patent leather.

7   See your doctor frequently.

## SWELLING

Swollen feet can be a signal for you to see your doctor. If you have a cardiac disorder, your feet may swell as the day wears on. If you press your thumb into the swelling and the indentation remains, this might indicate heart trouble. Kidney problems may also disturb the metabolism, manifested by swollen hands or feet. Sometimes swollen feet may indicate liver problems, or simply be a side-effect of an oral contraceptive. There may be only a minor vascular disorder. When the blood passing through the arteries and returning via the veins may get trapped in the foot, the tissues will swell. In any event, consult your doctor for the correct diagnosis.

There are other, simpler, causes of swollen feet. Garters, tight garments, temperature change in warmer weather, even crossed legs may interfere with regular blood flow. Sodium retention in the system may also be responsible and often affects women before the menstrual period. In this case, hormonal changes cause the tissues to retain a greater amount of sodium and water; you can reduce your salt intake to minimize this reaction. Diuretics are often prescribed for premenstrual sodium retention as a palliative.

## Varicose Veins

When the valves in the superficial veins of the leg are not working properly, blood cannot circulate freely and will back up. These veins are then said to be "varicosed," or swollen, because the blood isn't moving in any direction. Also, since the blood is not moving, the skin becomes discolored, often turning either blue or brown. The blood becomes stagnant and may even clot. Circulation is fighting a losing battle against gravity in this case and the heart just cannot seem to pump the blood flow upward. Whenever gravity enters the picture, such as during prolonged walking or standing, the foot responds by slowly swelling; and just as slowly the swelling will abate later, once you are seated. Varicose veins are an occupational hazard for beauticians, salespeople, restaurant workers, or any people who have to stay on their feet for hours on end, minimizing the blood's chance to return upward. If your occupation requires standing, it would be wise to keep your feet up during coffee breaks and after work. Since your feet provide your livelihood, you had best take care of them.

The additional weight of pregnancy will take its toll on the feet; swelling or varicose veins may appear. But since these conditions are the result of temporary inactivity and added weight, they will disappear once normal activity is resumed. Elevating your feet— even in bed—may be helpful during pregnancy. It is important to keep up your walking, but in a sturdy shoe with the lowest, broadest heel and a wide toe box. You can't afford to totter about on high heels right now. Good foot function is imperative and comfort is the best incentive. Within six weeks after childbirth, your feet should return to their former size and varicose veins will probably just as quickly disappear.

In order to keep varicose veins at bay, try to outwit gravity by keeping the circulation moving. Muscles will then massage the blood flow into action. For people with varicose veins, especially women during pregnancy, elastic support hosiery will help the blood to return upward to the heart. Elevating your feet above the heart level will also encourage the blood to reach the heart. Simple exercises such as moving your ankle in a circle above your head or spelling out the alphabet with your feet raised will help, too.

The removing of varicose veins by surgery is generally considered a cosmetic process. If your doctor feels that the deeper veins can permanently work overtime, he or she may operate on the superficial veins by transferring their function to their stronger neighbors.

If your varicose vein condition is severe, the doctor may elect to strip the veins. The ancient Greek medical sage Galen was the first to perform the stripping technique in the second century B.C. The surgeon makes two or more incisions, usually at the ankle, and passes a vein stripper through the long superficial vein in the leg; this vein is then pulled out through the incisions. Almost all the varicose veins are thereby removed and blood circulation will probably improve. This procedure means a one- to three-day hospital visit and about three weeks of leg supports, such as sturdy support hose, which do not hamper walking. Pain is minimal.

If your doctor decides to save the varicose vein by sealing off the part that is not working well, injection therapy is generally required. A hardening agent is injected into the damaged vein and the leg is then bandaged for six weeks. If the compression is effective, blood flow will be diverted to other veins and should be stimulated.

Both treatments are considered expedient by most doctors and have shown satisfactory results in various surveys. Once you discover which veins are not doing their job, you and your doctor can decide on the proper course of action.

## Footsteps to Health

> *"You can't stay young
> if you're not walking properly."*
> DR. ELIZABETH ROBERTS

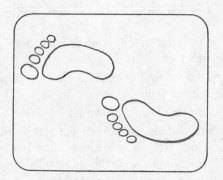

Since human nature prompts us to overlook problems until they stare us in the face, preventive measures are difficult to incorporate into our daily routines. Too often it is too late to do anything yourself once you notice that something is wrong. Our consciousness doesn't seem to encompass the condition of our feet, and we may suffer from this oversight after age twenty-five.

Dr. Elizabeth Roberts firmly believes that many older people allow their lives to be limited by their neglected feet, which just don't seem to want to carry on. If mandatory podiatry care could be integrated into the health programs at geriatric institutions, she feels, this would improve the quality of life for the elderly. "A person in a rest home may be too bashful to speak up about bad feet. Lack of exercise may then lead to other problems, and ultimately the person feels trapped by leaden feet," she explains. In a way, the foot acts as a barometer of the general state of the body. Anemia, arthritis, diabetes, circulation, and kidney disorders may all often be detected first in the feet.

But we don't have to be in a geriatric institution to know how it feels to be a prisoner of achy feet. The well-being of the foot is important at any age. As long as you treat those hardworking appendages with all due respect, they shouldn't let you down. Let common sense be your guide.

Good foot hygiene can be summarized in three general categories:

1   Cleanliness above all! Change hosiery and shoes every day, and if your feet perspire heavily, change your hosiery more often.

> Wash your feet carefully and dry thoroughly, especially between the toes.
>
> Allow your feet to "air out." Don't keep them locked up in shoes all the time.
>
> Trim your toenails straight across.
>
> Use creams to keep the skin supple and powders on your feet to absorb extra moisture and to prevent infection and odor. Knock out any accumulated powder in your shoes so that it will not gum up when combined with moisture.

2   Exercise! Keep your feet in shape by using them. You can do these movements at your desk or in an easy chair when reading or chatting or watching television: Simply rotate your foot to limber it up. For toning ligaments and tendons, try picking up marbles with your toes—even if only for a few minutes. Stretch your Achilles tendons and calf muscles by "tapping" them out—alternately tapping on the floor with your heels and toes from a sitting position. The heel cords will also benefit by standing and poising your toes on a telephone directory about 2

inches thick with your heel on the floor. Finish up your exercise regimen by "weight-lifting"—hanging a pocketbook or other weight from each ankle and lifting it while sitting.

Additionally, Dr. Suzanne Levine of New York's Mt. Sinai Hospital recommends rope jumping to strengthen the feet and ankles in the comfort of your own home—assuming your downstairs neighbors don't object!

**3** Visit your doctor before any foot problem reaches emergency proportions. A regular check-up—such as that with your dentist—may mean walking easy for life.

# FOOT SAVERS

## Podiatry

Foot care has been a cultural concern through the ages, as evidenced by the Egyptian Papyrus Ebers, circa 1500 B.C., which contains the earliest written remedies for foot care problems. These ancient antidotes had been compiled from even earlier times. Hikesios of Smyrna is credited with fashioning the first corn plaster around 100 B.C. The early Greek physicians Hippocrates and Galen, of the fifth and second centuries B.C. respectively, both wrote extensively on the feet in their learned works.

More organized legions of foot experts appeared much later, alongside surgeons and dentists, in the medieval guilds of barber surgeons. It was not until 1774 that chiropody, the direct ancestor of podiatry, made its debut. A treatise appeared by a D. Low in London that year entitled *Chiropodolgia: A Scientific Enquiry in the Cause of Corns, Warts, etc.* that made a big splash. Following this publication, a Dr. Lyons in London applied for a license to practice on feet; simultaneously self-proclaimed "corncutters" were

Ye Olde Foote

cropping up in America. For 25 cents, a local barbershop promised to put an end to corn discomfort—perhaps more a pedicure than a truly surgical procedure, but effective nonetheless.

By 1840 the first podiatric office opened in Boston under the aegis of Dr. Nehemiah Kenison. That same year he and two relatives treated the feet of workers in the New England textile and shoe factories, thereby building up a solid clientele. Another pioneer in the field, Dr. Isacaar Zacharie, treated President Abraham Lincoln's tired feet.

In 1895 New York State initiated a move to elevate the non-professional art of chiropody to a licensed professional practice by an act of the legislature. But it wasn't until 1912 that the National Association of Chiropodists convened in Chicago with representatives from thirteen states. Twenty-five years later, chiropody was a licensed profession throughout the United States, Canada, the United Kingdom, Australia, and New Zealand. The term "podiatry" was coined in 1917 and became the official successor to "chiropody" in 1958 when the National Association of Chiropodists changed its name to the American Podiatry Association.

Since 1958 great strides have been made in American podiatry. The prepodiatry program is now identical to that of its premed and predentistry counterparts. The majority of students require eight years of schooling—four in premedical study and four years of podiatric medicine—to earn a degree as Doctor of Podiatric Medicine (D.P.M.). Technically, three years of undergraduate work will suffice but B.A.s are preferred. One year of internship and between one to three years of residency generally follow this course of study. With the prevalence of neglected feet, the demand for skilled specialists seems never to wane; although the number of podiatry graduates has doubled since 1966, the needs of foot sufferers still cannot be met. Statistics show that each year there are about 28 million patient visits made to podiatrists. As of 1979, for every 670 people there was one medical doctor and for every 2,000, one dentist, in contrast to one podiatrist for every 23,-000 people and 46,000 feet! The 7,500-plus men and women licensed to treat feet have had to pass stiff tests in the states in which they choose to practice. And, in return, they earn an average of $42,000 a year (1979 figure).

In 1979, there were five accredited American podiatry schools, in San Francisco, Chicago, Cleveland, Philadelphia, and New York City. Plans for new schools are presently on the drawing boards. Each school is accredited by the Council on Podiatric Education. The four-year intensive program covers the basic sciences and ultimately clinical experience of up to three years. All conditions of foot malfunction are studied, as a complement to the skills of the M.D. who specializes in areas other than feet. Later on, the podiatry student may choose to specialize in surgery, podopediatrics, podogeriatrics, podiatric sports medicine, or biomechanics. The American training program is more rigorous than that of any other country. Foot specialists abroad may simply do a course of study for six months with a company such as that manufacturing Dr. Scholl's brand products. But as interest in the foot increases, information will become more accessible and the quality of foot care will improve around the world.

Keeping abreast of new developments is particularly important in the medical field since new ground is constantly being broken. New York State, for instance, has instituted a mandatory continuing education program among podiatrists. Every second year, when the D.P.M. is required to reregister for a license, a certain number of credits must be earned in approved areas; although the doctor is free to reject new methods, it is important at least to be exposed to the material.

Most up-to-date is the branch of podiatry known as "ambulatory surgery." The running battle between podiatrists and orthopedists for hospital space forced many podiatrists to resort to office surgery. In this way, simple disorders could be permanently corrected in an office visit and the patient could walk out a bit numbed but looking forward to happier feet.

## Self-massage

Whether you have formal training in massage or not, we all know of the comforting sensation that a massage has on a sore muscle. Rubbing the achy area is almost an involuntary reaction. The earliest record of massage—known as *an-ma*—dates back to about 2700 B.C. in China. Greeks and Romans both prescribed the use of massage in the *gymnasia*, encouraged by the enthusiasm of Hippocrates and Galen. In India the Laws of Manu were devised to formalize technique. The Middle Ages in the West then cast massage aside, classifying it as folklore medicine, and until the nineteenth century it was almost completely disregarded. Now, although its beneficial results are acknowledged, doctors are still not sure how massage works—except that it eases tense muscles that are responsible for pain.

In 1812 a Swedish teacher of gymnastics, Pehr Henrik Ling, revived the use of massage by applying it more scientifically to the anatomy. He outlined the different manipulations: *effleurage*—a long rhythmical stroke; *pétrissage,* or *foulage*—kneading; friction—small circular movements; *tapotement*—a percussive movement;

vibration—a trembling gesture. The warm, soothing effect produced by massaging the skin's nerve endings relaxes and stimulates the body. Circulation improves while noxious substances are flushed out; perspiration is one way to release these. Swelling in the joints may lessen as blood rushes back to the heart and the lymph flow is stimulated. Ligaments and tendons also benefit. In fact, Swedish massage is said to be as beneficial to the whole body as a good long walk.

If your feet are strained from overexertion or prolonged standing, a foot massage will help to revitalize them. Muscles will feel renewed as circulation speeds up. If you massage your feet on a regular basis, some of your foot troubles may fade—and perhaps problems in remote parts of the body as well. Muscle tone, pulse, and respiration should all improve as a vigorous massage helps dispel toxic substances. If you don't have the time or patience for a foot massage, simply roll a golf ball under each longitudinal arch to loosen and limber up the feet. You don't even have to remove your hosiery and you can exert as much pressure as you need.

The only times you should avoid a foot massage are if you have any sign of fever, infection, hemorrhage, phlebitis, thrombosis, varicose veins, fracture, jaundice, or any type of tumor. In the case of body infection, a foot massage may cause it to spread to a greater area. With such disorders as phlebitis and thrombosis, a foot massage may dislodge the blood clot and cause it to move to the heart, which could be fatal. Pregnant women should only be massaged under the supervision of a doctor. Never massage directly after a meal since it will divert the blood from the digestive system where it is needed.

For a thorough foot massage, make yourself comfortable; recline if you like or prop up your back and shoulders. Choose a lubricant—either a commercial hand cream or a vegetable oil. Coconut and safflower oils are among the most effective lubricants according to the Chinese; the latter is said to improve the body flow of energy. Take your time so as to allow your feet to enjoy all the possible benefits.

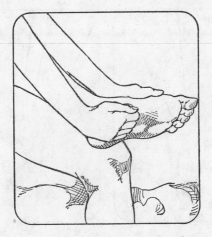

Follow these steps for each foot:

**1**  Lubricate your foot lightly and work the oil into the sole with your closed fist. Allow your fist knuckles to outline circles from top to bottom.

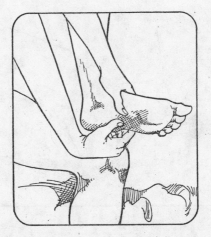

**2**  Open your hand and circle the sole with your thumbs. On the heel and ankle area, use all your fingers.

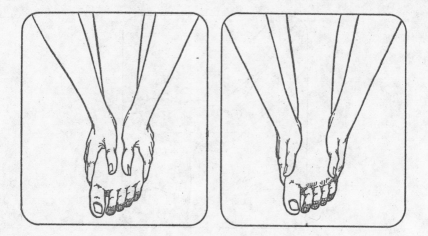

**3** Now take hold of your foot with both hands, fingertips on the sole and thumbs on top. Press firmly; then slide the thumbs down to the edge of the sole. Repeat once.

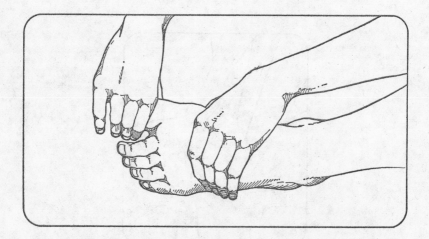

**4** Hold the big toe with your index finger and thumb. Gently pull and allow your fingers to slide off. Do this for all the toes.

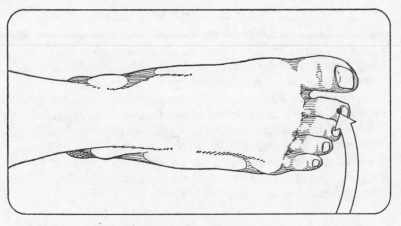

Massage point for hangover cure.

Massage aficionados believe that manipulating the body, especially the feet, can cure a wide range of ills if applied correctly. So you might try the following antidotes popular in the Orient for these relatively common woes. (But think of these measures as first aid—to provide temporary relief, if any.)

*Hangover:* Hold your second toes firmly with your thumb and forefinger. Press the base of the toenail on each foot where it emerges from the matrix. Use a pinching motion, applying as much pressure as you can tolerate.

*Insect bite:* Press your thumb on the outer edge of each foot just behind the toe knuckle of the little toe to relieve pain.

*Sunburn:* Press your thumb on the outer edge of each foot just above the fifth toe knuckle; apply as much pressure as feels comfortable.

## Alternate Routes

With interest in health maintenance on the rise, many people are beginning to educate themselves as to the alternate methods of treatment. Foot care is no exception. The movement toward investigation of alternate treatments is only in the early stages and still requires further research by the medical profession. However, if properly administered by a licensed practitioner, some complaints may find relief in acupuncture, shiatsu, or reflexology. These treatments cannot be self-administered but require a qualified professional. Contact the American Medical Association or ask your podiatrist for recommendations of practitioners in your area.

Since podiatrists are best qualified to treat the problems of feet, the person with a foot disorder should enlist their expertise before consulting the alternate routes. As well-informed consumers, however, it is important to be aware of all developments in the field of foot care, such as the following methods.

## ACUPUNCTURE

> *"Wind, rain, cold, and heat, unless they find the body weak cannot by themselves do injury to man."*
>
> LING SHU

As the gap between Eastern and Western medicine closes, more and more Americans may be considering acupuncture as a medical alternative. This "new" way to heal ailments via the insertion of very fine needles into specific body points is 5,000 years old, yet it was only introduced to the West in the mid-twentieth century. Mainland China has at least 1 million acupuncture specialists, including over 150,000 who are also M.D.s; in Japan there are about 50,000 acupuncturists. Only between 2,000 and 3,000 serve the entire Western world, with a mere handful in the U.S. where licenses to practice legally are required in every state.

There is no acupuncture institute in the U.S., but Britain has a College of Chinese Acupuncture, which was established in 1961, for professional training. A diploma from this school, of course, is not a license to practice in the United States. But interest in the ancient treatment is fast gaining in the U.S., where the World Acupuncture Congress of 1974 was held, in Philadelphia.

What is acupuncture and how can the body heal itself when used as a pincushion? Although these questions nag the skeptical

Western mind, credit must be given to a method of healing that has survived the millennia. Basic Chinese medical principles were codified for general use in a famous handbook written in about 400 B.C., *Nei Ching* (*The Yellow Emperor's Classic of Internal Medicine*). In the handbook the methods and theory of acupuncture are described and analyzed. After this information became generally available, a great number of Chinese cultivated healing skills and developed an interest in acupuncture. These "barefoot doctors" of rural China began to cater to community needs when epidemics hit, perhaps practicing on their own families to sharpen their abilities.

Traditionally, the acupuncturist has three goals: to treat the mind and body as a single entity; to seek the underlying problem; and to remove the immediate discomfort. Manual dexterity is essential in an acupuncturist and requires considerable practice to attain.

Acupuncture today is administered by means of stainless steel needles about the diameter of a hair strand. Formerly, needles were handmade of bone, but unbreakable modern materials are preferable. There is almost no pain involved and often the patient experiences no sensation whatsoever. The more relaxed the patient feels, the less likely he or she will be to feel anything at all. Needles range in length from ½ inch to 4 inches. In most cases, they are inserted just below the skin's surface but may be pressed up to 3 inches deep. No matter how far in the needles are, the patient feels the same sensation, which simply depends on the pain threshold of the individual. The feeling has been described as dull and deep, tingling, or just a vague pinch. Usually three to eight needles are required. Treatment lasts an average of half an hour. The practitioner slightly stretches the patient's skin with one hand while inserting the needle in a clockwise, twirling motion with the other. The needles are placed in specified parts of the body and no blood is drawn; there should be no infection since the needles are sterilized.

Often the needles are inserted into the feet and lower legs, which serve as a "map" of all the internal organs. The area between the knees and toes is thought to contain a series of points (*tsubos*) which relate to every other part of the body. For example, a point in the toe may relieve a headache, another point intestinal problems. To the acupuncturist, the human body is a highly complex electrical circuit containing twelve channels that run its full length. Chinese medical theory stipulates that the life force (*ch'i,* pronounced "key") controls the proper functioning of the body the way fuel keeps a car going. This force travels through the organs via the twelve channels, or meridians. When the flow is obstructed, illness results. When the acupuncturist applies needles to the corresponding trouble spots, energy can either be released or induced until balance is regained.

Some patients claim that acupuncture applied to the feet is an effective birth control method! However, the use of acupuncture for this purpose is not condoned by general practitioners of Western medicine.

Despite the lack of scientific explanation, there is evidence that in some cases acupuncture has worked. Recent tests show that the needles may stimulate receptors that send messages to the brain and prompt the release of endorphins. The endorphins then circulate in the body like hormones and block the pain pathways; these morphinelike peptide molecules have an analgesic effect on the central nervous system. The Acupuncture Research Project at UCLA has reported that acupuncture may become a viable alternative to surgery, and in the light of this new information the option for patients may come sooner than we think.

## SHIATSU

Literally, *shiatsu* translates from Japanese as "finger pressure." It has developed from 4,000 years of Oriental medicine as a hybrid of acupuncture and *an-ma* massage. There are at least 20,000 licensed *shiatsu* therapists in Japan today working with the same principles as do acupuncturists—only without needles.

According to *shiatsu* theory, the foot contains important nerve endings from all over the body, so that body ailments are mirrored in the foot: foot massage as treatment is therefore considered effective. The sole is a miniature model of the human anatomy: the toes relate to the head, eyes, ears and nose; the ball of the foot to the solar plexus organs (liver, gall bladder, pancreas); the area under the longitudinal arch to the kidneys and small intestine; the area under the heel to the sex organs. Excessive pain in any part of the foot is thought to indicate disorder in the corresponding part of the body.

*Shiatsu* practitioners allege that by using your fingers in a certain manner, you can treat your illnesses yourself. Self-*shiatsu*, developed recently by Tokujiro Namikoshi, is based on the premise that touch can improve physical well-being as well as cure ailments. Oriental doctors believe that the degeneration associated with aging begins in the legs, so it is most important to take good care of that region.

Although only a *shiatsu* specialist can perform complicated massages, it is claimed that you can learn to use it to wake up tired feet yourself. By loosening muscles, you increase your blood flow and thus reduce the accumulation of lactic acid, often blamed for muscle aches. When massaging your feet according to *shiatsu* rules, always press down with the ball of the thumb, not the tip, and exert pressure for five to seven seconds. For covering a wider span, use both thumbs together.

Self-*shiatsu* is best when you are sitting in a chair. For a complete *shiatsu* foot massage, put your feet on the floor. The points you will knead are located between the tendons, in the recesses. Place your thumbs together in the depression located about two inches behind the web space formed by the first two toes of the foot you are working on. Important points that connect to other parts of the body are found in these "ditches" between the tendons that lead to the toes.

1  Press for three seconds and pause.

2  Moving thumbs from the midfoot toward the toes, repeat this pressure for three seconds and pause again.

3  Repeat this procedure from the "ditch" in the midfoot toward each toe.

To refresh your toes, cross the right leg over the left and grab the big right toe, with your left thumb on top and index finger beneath. Squeeze for about three seconds. Repeat at the joint of the big toe and finally pinch the toe by squeezing it from both sides.

The sole of the foot contains four pressure points, according to *shiatsu* practice. The first three are on the lengthwise midline and the fourth is toward the back of the longitudinal arch (also known as the "valley of the sole"). Pressing each of these points with both thumbs working from top to bottom is supposed to relieve fatigue and insomnia.

In New York State, *shiatsu* is recognized as a medical technique and can only be performed legally by doctors. But the sentiment behind it, as expressed by Tokujiro Namikoshi, has sifted down through the years: "The heart of *shiatsu* is like pure maternal affection; the pressure of the hands causes the springs of life to flow."

## REFLEXOLOGY

> "*There is only one disease, physical or mental,
> and its name is congestion.*"
> EUNICE INGHAM, "STORIES THE FEET HAVE TOLD"

Ancient teachings claim that the feet stand as a map of man's physical state. By protecting our feet in shoes, the theory goes, we preserve the integrity of this map and make it easier for the reflexologist to "read" the body by scanning the feet. Foot-zone therapy —known now as "reflexology"—uses ancient Chinese thought in a new way. In the days before shoes, the sole of the foot was naturally massaged by stones and pebbles underfoot which stimulated the circulation and dispersed waste material that settled at the bottom of the body. Now we must use our hands to achieve the same ends.

In 1913 Dr. William Fitzgerald first introduced his version of reflexology to the United States. He divided the body into ten longitudinal zones, each containing separate nerve stimulation patterns corresponding to the organs within its perimeters and having corresponding zones in the foot. If a gland or organ overlapped into two zones, treatment involved both zones of the foot. Most helped by this method, he claimed, would be the internal organs. By rubbing the appropriate zones, or "reflex points," on the foot,

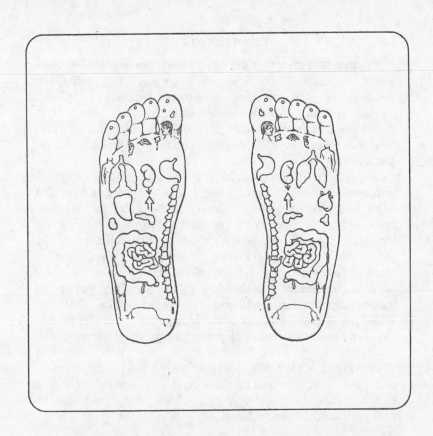

the corresponding parts of the body would be renewed and internal cleanliness would be restored. Natural sediment which settles in the feet would be brushed away and pain would be relieved, according to Dr. Fitzgerald.

Touch, he claimed, releases an electric-nerve impulse which in turn stimulates the body—although there are no anatomical connections between these reflexes and the internal organs. The central principle is that the body works as an electromechanism able to short-circuit at any time and disturb the function of the inner workings. Foot problems mean organ malfunctions, Dr. Fitzgerald surmised. Taking this theory further, he decided that therapeutic massage of the corresponding area of the sole would promote internal healing.

However, in reflexology massage alone is not enough. Dr. Fitzgerald recommended modification in other areas such as diet. His principles were later documented by two of his disciples, Mildred Carter and Eunice Ingham. Carter's book, *Helping Yourself With Reflexology,* outlines the basic philosophy, while Ingham's work, *Stories the Feet Have Told,* offers practical examples and case histories.

In treating a friend's feet, Carter suggests a comfortable, seated arrangement since the process may last as long as one hour. To begin, she recommends your examining the soles for any irritation and try to avoid these sore spots. Then proceed to the solar plexus point directly beneath the ball of the foot, along the second metatarsal, using thumb pressure in a rolling, circular motion. This pressure is said to relieve stray tension. Toes are next and then move your hand down the foot from outside to inside. Alternate feet while you massage to maintain balance. When you discover a tender spot, massage for about one minute and then return to it later. The greater the pressure, the better the results are thought to be.

In her book, Carter points out that many massages may be necessary until effects become manifest. So if your longitudinal arches hurt, according to reflexology, don't blame your shoes: look to your intestines for the problem!

# BEST FOOT FORWARD

## Getting Your Feet Wet

Soaking one's feet evokes luxurious images. After her bath, Cleopatra is said to have had her slaves massage scented oils into her feet which were then fanned with peacock feathers. Today, European health spas feature modern variations on this theme, often using herbal bath additives. Many in the medical field question this technique—they point out that the foot is waterproof and therefore the herbal bath is useless and a waste of money. Plain hot water, these skeptics claim, is just as effective. Still, there is no harm in trying out the herbal "decoctions" recorded since at least 2700 B.C., according to Chinese documents—and it smells great. Turn your bathroom into an exclusive health resort by investing in a few simple supplies.

First of all you will need a basin or tub in which to rest your feet and legs to midcalf. Even a pail will do. Fifteen minutes a day will provide welcome relief even if you can't undo a lifetime's damage with this brief treatment. Ideally, basic health

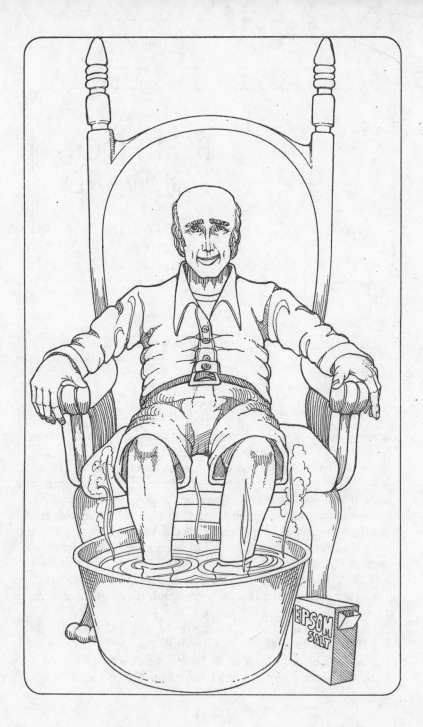

care of the foot calls for two daily baths, an alcohol rubdown, powdering, and gentle massage. If you have access to a whirlpool bath, five minutes will suffice to relax your feet and stimulate blood flow. For the more experimental, choose the appropriate herbal decoction, listed below, for your troubled feet. Wrap a few ounces of the substance in a cloth bag (an old clean sock will do) and boil it in a quart of water or so. Simply pour the water into your foot tub or—the lazy person's method—just hang the bag over the hot-water tap and allow the water to run through it tea-bag style. Then use the bag as a washcloth on your feet for sweet-smelling results.

### Cold Feet

Steep 3 to 4 ounces of mustard powder in a warm footbath. Besides warming the feet, this bath helps clear head colds, according to one old wives' tale.

If your feet are chronically cold and chilblains (swollen, red toes) develop, the following added to your footbath may relieve discomfort: barberry, oat, or sage. Add one of these herbs to your footbath water daily. Also suggested by ancient sources is rosemary, for improving the circulation; one medieval belief considers this herb an effective measure against aging.

### Corns and Calluses

Helpful bath ingredients are said to be lemon and camomile. Camomile can be used in tea-bag form, that is, simply soaking the bag in the footbath. Marigold flower soap is also supposed to help soften the skin.

### Cramps

Steep 3 to 4 ounces of loose thyme in a bag in 1 pint of boiling water for 10 minutes. Pour this into a warm footbath.

### Disco Fatigue

For all-night dancer's swollen feet, podiatrists recommend that you soak feet in water and ice cubes.

## Dry Skin

Doctors suggest that Vitamin A or D cream may be effective.

## Gout

Steep a teabag of comfrey in hot tap water and add to footbath.

## Perspiring Feet

Camomile is reputed to be a reliable antidote for this condition. Also considered effective are dried walnut leaves. Boil 1 pound of these leaves in 1½ quarts of water for 45 minutes and pour into footbath.

## Softness of Feet

If your feet are too soft, try an old boxer's trick and soak them in a solution of warm water and rock salt. Fighters do this to their hands to build up knuckle resistance.

## Tired Feet

To revitalize beat-up feet, try a cold footbath until you either can't take it any more or your feet warm up. Alternating hot and cold dowses (1 to 2 minutes in hot water, then ½ minute in cold) for 15 minutes may be most helpful. End this treatment on a cold-water note. If you feel ambitious, place pebbles in the bottom of your footbath and press your feet against them to stimulate circulation. A vigorous alcohol rubdown or a cider vinegar soak should prove equally invigorating.

For an *après bain* rubdown, use a mixture of camphorated oil liniment and sweet almond oil in equal parts. Or, for those who prefer quick gratification, a cooling menthol cream with soothing lanolin should do.

## Varicose Veins

Barberry, sassafras, sweet marjoram, and witch hazel in one's bath are old standbys in medical folklore. Fern rootstock is also said to have favorable results; boil 1 pound in water and add to your bath. Rootstock was considered a good luck charm in the Middle Ages; if one trimmed off all but five fronds of the branch, it looked like a hand trying to ward off evil spirits.

## Warts

One old remedy calls for lemon in any amount, mixed to taste, diluted into your footbath water.

If you're looking for an aromatic foot refresher, try mixing lavender, rose petals, and camomile with equal parts of borax and orris-root powder. Gentian by itself also makes an appealing footbath.

For the most in sensual footbaths, combine the following in equal parts: corn poppy, early-flowering periwinkle, fragrant valerian, maidenhair male fern, and pansy. Add 1 ounce of this potion to 1 quart of water and boil. Simmer for a few minutes and then steep for about ½ hour. Strain and add to your footbath.

As an appropriate finale to this ultimate experience, anoint your delicately scented pedal extremities with the juice of fresh-squeezed lemons to close the pores. Besides smelling good, lemons will combat any stray fungal matter that might threaten the well-being of your exhilarated feet.

## Foot Fantastic

> *"At the dinner table the lover will lose no opportunity*
> *for establishing secret contact between the hands*
> *and the feet of his mistress."*
>
> OVID

Many people mistakenly regard feet as the least attractive part of the body, not realizing their latent qualities. To hide them in shoes is no solution, any more than high-necked blouses or baggy trousers can conceal the underlying truths. You'll have to face your feet one of these days. And when you do, you may discover that they have more potential for beauty than you ever gave them credit for. George du Maurier recognized this potential for beauty in his novel *Trilby,* about an artist's model whose greatest assets were her delicate and provocative feet. After all, you lean on them all the time—why not treat them with respect and affection?

Mentally list all the irregularities of your feet: Do you have calluses, corns, or other lumps? Are any of your toenails blackened? Are you one of the notorious nail-pickers known to abuse the fifth toe?

After you eliminate the obvious villains—such as pinching shoes —a thorough self-administered pedicure may be sufficient to keep your other problems at bay. Both men and women can benefit from giving themselves pedicures. And if you take the time to repeat this ritual once a month, your feet should be in good shape. As Dr. Jonathan Zizmor says, a pedicure will make you feel good, because when your feet are happy, so is your disposition.

In order to give yourself a proper pedicure, you will need a basic foot-improvement kit: a small plastic pail, a nail clipper, an emery board, an orange stick, a small nail brush, petroleum jelly or hand cream, and a pumice stone.

Mimi Glaser, a professional pedicurist at an elegant salon in New York City, suggests this procedure for best results:

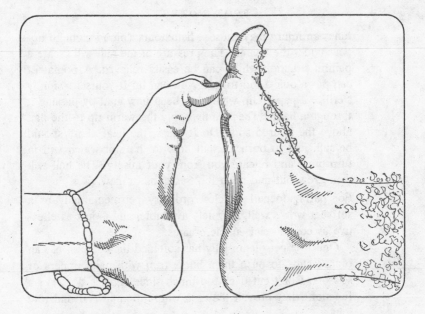

1 Wash your feet thoroughly. For those hard-to-reach places, apply a pasty mixture of baking soda and water with a brush or washcloth. Scrub and rinse feet.

2 For a quick soak, add a mild shampoo or dish-washing liquid to warm water and allow your feet to relax in it. For an extra lift, add Epsom salts or massage your feet first with cider vinegar. Skin and toenails will then be soft and pliable.

3 When toenail clipping, never round off the nail—that may lead to ingrown infections. Simply clip the nails straight across—"sparingly," implores Mimi. Gently clip off any slivers of dead skin around the nail. Use the emery board to smooth the nail edge. Your object is a clean, healthy toenail.

Tennis players especially seem to develop toenail infections and should be most careful about cleaning their feet after a match. The big toe bears the brunt of the game and should be protected by a thin layer of lamb's wool. Sometimes an injury may cause a hematoma (blood clot) to appear under the toenail. The pressure of the nail will create a painful situation which can be easily relieved. A podiatrist can put a quick end to it or you can do it yourself. Simply sterilize a paper clip which has been unwound by passing it through a flame. Then gently apply the warm tip to the nail above the injured spot. Don't press; the heat alone should be sufficient to burn a small hole to the clot which will in turn burst and release you from your misery. The nail will then grow out and soon look as good as new.

4   For paring toenail cuticles, ordinary petroleum jelly as a softener works well, is widely available, and is just as effective as commercial cuticle creams.

Once the petroleum jelly has softened the cuticles, use an orange stick to push them back; trim with nail clippers or scissors. Don't cut back too much since cuticles do serve a function: they protect the area where the nail and nail fold join.

5   Return your feet to the basin for another soak. Wet the pumice stone and rub against callused areas. If you are rubbing too hard, you will know since your foot will grow unbearably warm. Take it easy for best results. Use the stone in smooth, sandinglike movements. If a pumice stone is too abrasive, use a nonmedicated polyester sponge to help reduce calluses. Or use a chiropody sponge or a simple loofah. By using these daily, you will keep calluses at a minimum. If calluses are your main problem, you might use salicylic acid soap for best results.

For those who prefer electricity to man power, battery-operated manicure/pedicure machines will also work off the layers of dead skin. Some have attachments for fingernails, toenails, calluses, and buffing. Be very careful if you use one since any cut into healthy skin may lead to infection. If there is any sign of infection, apply a disinfectant—particularly on any sign of ingrown toenails.

If you have a lot of time on your hands, spend it on your feet. For permanent softening of stubborn calluses, cream your feet and tie plastic bags around them. Sit with legs elevated to improve circulation and stimulate body heat to absorb cream. After half an hour, unwrap and pumice the calluses.

6  Once your feet are completely dried, massage them with your favorite hand cream or petroleum jelly, from the toes up to the heels. The late Duke of Windsor, it is said, treated his feet to the best face creams. But if applied sparingly and massaged thoroughly, simple petroleum jelly is as effective as a sweeter-smelling (and far more expensive) moisturizer.

7  Now use an astringent on your feet to tighten the pores. Mimi uses cider vinegar. Rubbing alcohol will do the trick, too; witch hazel is also a relaxing way to wind up the pedicure.

For women who like colorful toenails, polish may now be applied. You can make this into an intimate ritual with your mate. In the film *Lolita,* Humbert Humbert capitalized on stolen moments with Lolita by administering a long and loving pedicure to his little darling. Toenail painting takes on a whole new light once it becomes a team effort.

This procedure is easy. First, separate your toes with tissue or cotton balls, whichever you prefer. Paint a base coat and two on top, making certain that the nail is fully covered—even paint a bit over the front edge to the underside. Then touch up with a finishing coat of clear polish. Dr. Zizmor, for one, regards all nail polishes as equal, so don't let fancy packaging dazzle you: the product is basically the same in any bottle.

Toe rings are catching on. Extend your erogenous zones to include your feet and live out the "bells on his/her fingers and rings on his/her toes" fantasy wherever you go.

Foot fetishism has been a ticklish matter by definition. But it may just be another exciting way to approach our sexuality. Think of it this way: you rub my foot, I'll rub yours. Since the foot is so well encased in our heavy shoes during the day, it retains a certain sensitivity when bare which makes it more ticklish and responsive than other parts of the anatomy. Groucho Marx's biographer, Charlotte Chandler, writes: "After 'You Bet Your Life,' Groucho often enjoyed his favorite indulgence, one that his mother had also enjoyed: nurse Happy tickled his feet." Definitely stepping into another dimension here. . . .

Middle European folklore has preserved an alleged aphrodisiac formula over the years for men, which calls for anointing the big toe with a mixture of Spanish fly and vegetable oil. This ritual is said to guarantee virility, since the big toe is considered a phallic symbol. The German psychologist Dr. G. Aigremont writes: "The naked foot exists as a means of sexual charming. There is a close connection between the foot and things sexual." In Slovenian the expression *"tretja noga"* (third foot) refers blatantly to the penis. And the eighteenth-century libertine Casanova remarked that men with sexual appetites equal to his felt a marked attraction to the female foot.

Once your foot is limber and supple, you might want to experiment with pedic lovemaking. After all, the feet were once "hands" and are therefore endowed with similar sensibilities. Excitement felt "down to the tips of your toes" is no exaggeration—the foot is a sensitive tactile organ. The Indian art of lovemaking included a toe kiss administered by a woman to her lover as a kicking off point.

It is widely accepted that the feet are affected by sexual activity. The renowned sex researcher Alfred Kinsey notes that after the obvious manifestations of arousal, the "next most noticeable . . . involve the feet and the toes. The toes of most individuals become curled or, contrariwise, spread when there is erotic arousal." Japanese erotic art featured curled toes for more than eight centuries as a symbolic representation of sexual response.

As you delve more deeply into the possibilities of your versatile feet, you may decide to join the Lotus Love Foot Erotica Club of America, an exclusive group of foot lovers. Spas designed for foot enthusiasts are found the world over if you have the persistence to sniff them out. Foot fetishists come out of the closet: the world is at hand!

# FANCY FOOTWORK

## The Rigors of Ballet

The great ballet dancer Mikhail Baryshnikov's gravity-defying leap into the White House chandelier in 1978 appeared as natural as that of a deer across a country road; spellbound, the spectator could only follow each movement, not considering the consequent effects on the dancer's delicately arched feet. Even a fragile, 100-pound ballerina will land on her feet with a force three times her weight. The mind boggles at the discrepancy between the effect on the spectator of Baryshnikov's graceful landing and how it in fact registered on his toe bones. It is the seductive image of lithe bodies fluttering on stage that lures young dancers into the fold, undeterred by the prospect of wear and tear on unsuspecting feet.

Dr. Murray Weisenfeld, a New York podiatrist who treats members of the American Ballet Theater, wonders how dancers maintain their sunny dispositions despite all the foot pain they experience. The Institute for Sports Medicine in New York City recently ranked classical ballet among the top three of sixty sports studied in terms of body strain, along with football and hockey.

Pain tolerance among dancers seems unusually high, but their feet will pay in later life.

As the official doctor of the New York City Ballet, orthopedist Dr. William Hamilton considers the Darwinian "survival of the fittest" as the decisive factor that distinguishes pros from amateurs. Three or four classes a day take their toll on vulnerable bodies.

Success in the dance world demands specific qualities: natural ability, motivation, and dedication rank first, followed closely by physical attitude (supple feet and body, natural turnout—the degree feet point away from each other, good pelvic rotation, healthy knees), and good training for proper technique. Although an elongated second toe may present problems, this should not necessarily discourage anyone from pursuing a dancing career. A naturally high longitudinal arch might seem ideal, but the functional ideal is the square foot with a sturdy arch. Doctors indicate that the feet of many prima ballerinas are far from ideal, so don't lose heart.

A "good" foot, as opposed to a "bad" foot, is distinguished by natural mobility. For the female dancer, the instep must be flexible to permit a good pointe position—when the dancer is on toe. (Faulty pointe position will lead to overstrain of the tendons.) And a flexible foot absorbs weight more efficiently. Although the high longitudinal arch is attractive, it is a rigid structure and prone to stress fractures.

Troublemakers for all dancers include the flatfoot—too weak— and the narrow foot—a shaky base. Wide, square feet are most durable. Foot length is also a decisive factor. The longer the foot, the more probable that chronic strain will arise. And then there is that variable in foot size, ever changing with age because of the enormous amount of time a dancer spends on his or her feet.

Above all, a dancer needs a lucky star, to ensure good fortune and prevent accidents or injuries which might nip a budding career. However, one need not aspire to the heights of a stage career; ballet can be an enjoyable form of exercise, a means to developing poise and grace.

Beginners usually range in age from five to eleven. Since the young body is naturally flexible, there should not be too many

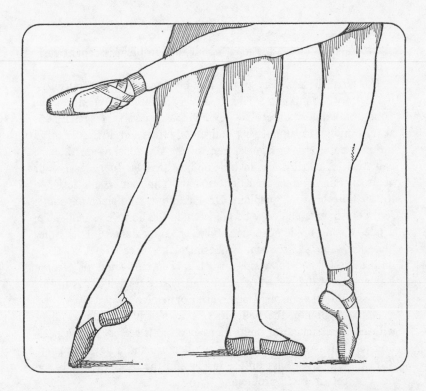

problems with this age group. A general looseness, characterized by loose hips and knees, will also mean good leg extension—but does not necessarily indicate loose feet. The constant up-and-down or in-and-out motions may cause foot stiffness. This may be connected to a weak subtalar joint, under the ankle; or it may be related to the instep. There is also the possibility of "tarsal coalition," which means that as the bones develop they do not separate properly. "Bars" of bone or cartilage will then form between the bones and hamper motion. Dance class will soon reveal this trouble, if pain does not alert the foot owner first.

Even the least dance-trained eye can recognize a dancer's posture. The feet turn outward—from the hip, not the knee. Research indicates that by age eight hip structure is permanently determined. Although exercises may improve the young dancer's turnout, pigeon toes may signify an abbreviated dancing career. Ice-skating and ballet classes may help if this problem is caught early on.

For girls, the next age group—roughly ages eleven to fourteen—begins work on pointe. This is a very exciting moment in the young ballerina's career. But until the youngster's musculature is strong enough to support her entire body, it is not advisable to go up on pointe. Ninety-five per cent of the lift depends on the two calf muscles which meet in the Achilles tendon. In general, four years of training must precede this step. "The foot wasn't designed to function this way," explains Dr. Hamilton. And since on-pointe foot adjustments can only be made while the bones are malleable, a late-starting novice can only hope to enjoy dance for its other pleasures after age sixteen. It doesn't make sense to get up there until the ability to follow through has been cultivated, as George Balanchine of the New York City Ballet likes to remark. And this time should come around age eleven or twelve.

Once on pointe, the ballerina's feet are truly in the spotlight with all their structural faults glaring—or so it seems. Pointe position relies heavily on good ankle architecture and a flexible instep. Stretching and working on the instep and the forefoot will lessen the chances of ankle problems.

Until permanent calluses have developed on the ball of the male dancer's foot and the tops of the toes for female dancers, soreness prevails. Meanwhile, inside the ball of the foot, the metatarsals are thickening because of the rigors of dance. When the stress on the foot is too much, stress fractures may result which means at least six weeks off the boards. The second metatarsal is often the unhappy victim of this injury, known as "Freiberg's infraction." Hairline fractures of the shafts of the second or third metatarsals occur as a result of recurrent impact and shock. Pain and swelling are the two major symptoms. Imagine a paper clip which is bent both ways over and over again—until something gives. Often even X-rays cannot reveal the subtle cracks, and given sufficient rest, healing may well precede a diagnosis. Jumping is taboo until the tenderness abates. In fact, rest is the only solution. Advanced fractures require splints and taping to assure proper mending.

The dancer's knee can be the victim of two disorders: Osgood-Schlatter disease ("choirboy's knee") and a hyperextended knee-cap ("trick knee"), which may mean the end to further dancing. The former condition afflicts the tendon connecting the kneecap to the front of the shinbone. Jumping, pliés (knee bends), and kneeling will aggravate this condition and cause tender masses to appear. Several months of rest may be prescribed, but by age sixteen, the dancer should have outgrown this syndrome. A trick knee is due to joint laxity, in which case the knee moves out of position and appears to lean backwards in an unnatural way. The dancer with a hyperextended knee must develop firm muscle control of the joint in order to keep it stable and avoid a "sway-kneed" posture.

The female dancer's feet begin to show the telltale marks of rigorous training between the ages of fourteen and eighteen. Bunions will appear but should not be removed until the dancer decides to retire. Bunions of this sort, as well as calluses, are good signs: they are Mother Nature's protection against the demands of dancing on pointe. Says one male pro: "To a dancer, bunions are beautiful. It's a matter of aesthetics and to a dancer it is a sign of hard work." In fact, some bunion is reasonably desirable since the toe box of the toe shoe rests against it in a "winged" foot configuration.

But for a dancer, surgery is not encouraged in the case of a bunion. Anything that might alter motion in the big-toe joint will affect the demipointe position which is not to be tampered with. The sesamoid bones under the big toes may become inflamed simply by the impact of jumping against a hard surface. Natural injuries restrict activity often enough without creating new causes for restriction.

The dancer's big toes take a beating each day and are often bruised. Jamming the big toes may cause bleeding under the nails or sprains. For obvious reasons, short toenails are the norm for dancers; they will thicken just as the bones have, because of the increase in pressure from above.

Rather than adjusting the structure of their feet, ballerinas seem to prefer that surgery be performed on their toe shoes. Since the mid-nineteenth century, specially designed toe shoes have been protecting talented feet the world over. Early toe dancers did not have this benefit and one hates to think what their feet looked like after a performance. Breaking in stiff, new toe shoes can be an obsessive pastime; rumor has it that they are smashed in doorways, pounded by hammers, and soaked in water until they lose their inherent stiffness. Some young dancers literally glue their tights onto the soles of their toe shoes to keep their feet securely in place and create appropriate arches according to personal taste, since there is no manufactured differentiation between the left and right slipper. The great Russian ballerina Anna Pavlova had her shoes broken in by a dancer with the same size foot to save herself this bother.

When the toe shoes are not sufficiently softened, their backs tend to irritate the ballerina's heels. Achilles bursitis often results, and is distinguished from Achilles tendinitis by examining the heel. Blisters may alert the ballerina to the abrasive shoe before bursitis sets in. By cutting the heels of their slippers and inserting wedges of elastic, dancers can get relief.

Injuries to the developing dancer's body heal fairly quickly, but once skeletal growth is complete, they will last much longer. Loose ligaments, tight muscles, or bone spurs may appear and interfere with performance. Foot and ankle injuries often weaken the original foot structure, and without proper exercises, complications are apt to result. The leading acute injury in ballet is the sprained ankle. Treatments range from rest to a cast worn for three to four weeks. Correct diagnosis by a physician is crucial if the ankle is to mend properly.

Another common dancer's complaint is tendinitis, the inflammation of a tendon. Because of stress, the fibers of leg tendons become damaged and swell. Rest and anti-inflammatory drugs are often prescribed by the physician, who also tries to determine the underlying causes. In a dancer, the most susceptible tendons are the Achilles tendon and the tendon between the big toe and the medial aspect of the ankle. The Achilles tendon may simply wear out like a piece of rope that is used over and over again in the same way. Experienced dancers know that in mild cases, warming the Achilles area will alleviate pain. Twenty minutes before practice sessions, a dancer should warm the area in a moist heat pack, then massage it with a mild liniment. Next, the foot should be wrapped in plastic and a woolen sock. After practice, ice or cold water should be applied for about twenty minutes.

Sometimes excessive pointe work will register in the ballerina's foot above the heel bone. "Dancer's heel" seems to be caused by inflammation, following injury, in the joint between the heel and the ankle. Pointing the foot will aggravate the pain, so pointe work should be limited. Again, rest is the best cure. But since most dancers swear by the German proverb "If I rest, I rust," dance activity should be limited and full pointe not attempted until discomfort abates.

Morton's neuroma, a knotting of nerve fibers, is also a common syndrome in female dancers, easily recognized by shooting pains extending from the web space on the ball of the foot between the metatarsals into the toes. A tight toe box or demipointe will aggravate the distressed nerves and minor surgery may be required. Another dancer's toe ailment—soft corns—may require surgical removal once they become chronic. Since these corns prefer a "tropical" climate, it is wise to keep feet dry at all times. Some dancers wrap their toes in brown paper to absorb excess moisture; lamb's wool is also a big favorite. Student dancers may even go so far as to wrap their toes in adhesive tape to keep them separated. This, however, is not professional practice, since performing dancers need to "feel" the floor for best results.

Most ballet injuries to both male and female dancers occur between 4 and 6 P.M., says Dr. Weisenfeld. By that time, after a day's practicing, mental fatigue has crept in and physical control has waned. Although practicing hard is an integral part of the dancer's life, it is important to recognize one's limits. While a dancer is waiting for an injury to heal, swimming is an apt exercise replacement: doing barre work in the water may add new dimensions to a dancer's experience. Professional dancers seem to rarely have serious foot problems; but perhaps this is due to their training which programs them to take everything in stride.

Of course, Nature may put in her two cents and arthritis will flare up, but some dancers manage to overcome this debilitating disease. Reliable sources allude to well-known dancers who have undergone joint-removal operations in the little toe, the flap of toe skin being then sewn onto the neighboring toe in a webbed configuration for foot stability. In most cases, however, doctors prefer to avoid this operation, which might jeopardize a dancer's career.

Although dancers are careful not to disturb the protective callus build-up on their feet, after pounding the boards all day long they find relief in foot soaks. Leading the list of soothing balms is Burow's solution, which acts as both an antiseptic and an astringent while dispersing heat effects. The dancer should avoid overuse of this solution since it may cause the skin to crack. Diluting it in the footbath or simply wrapping a towel soaked in the diluted solution about the foot and encasing it in plastic wrap are two ways to avoid skin irritations. If the skin becomes too hard, paint the foot daily with tincture of benzoin and cover with talc after it dries. Sometimes a hot-water foot soak with soap flakes may be just as effective.

# STEPPING LIVELY
## Running

*"There is no doubt that running
has elevated the status of the foot."*
DR. ELIZABETH ROBERTS

Except for a contemporary Rip Van Winkle and babes in arms, everyone knows of the running mania which has swept millions of the world's population off their feet in recent years. A conservative estimate is 30 million runners worldwide, with over one third in the U.S., some of whom are seriously afflicted with "marathon fever." Suddenly those already abused appendages we affectionately refer to as "tootsies," "dogs," or "dewbeaters" are expected to run sometimes as much as twenty miles a day, a distance which translates into 17,000 foot strikes against the ground, often against such uncongenial surfaces as concrete.

Minor foot discomfort when inflicted 17,000 times may give rise to major complications. As people become more and more passionately involved in sports, doctors find it futile to prescribe rest and immobility for their foot ailments. As the various "overuse" foot syndromes crop up, doctors have had to evolve new attitudes to explain and treat the heel spurs, tendinitis, shin splints,

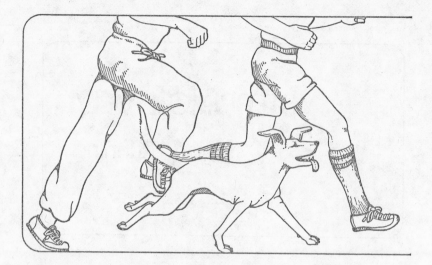

muscle pulls, and stress fractures that begin appearing after a runner logs more than thirty miles a week. When runners overdo, as the philosopher-podiatrist Dr. Richard Schuster explains, "The body begins to break down. It's like an old jalopy, good enough to get you to the supermarket but if you try to run it in the Grand Prix, it'll fall apart."

And so "sports medicine" was born in the early 1970s as an innovative and important sub-specialty, under the combined aegis of the American Medical Association and the American Academy of Podiatry. Before this running mania took hold, sports medicine was restricted to a sort of "first aid for athletes"; afterward, it evolved into a new type of preventive medicine, with podiatry as an ancillary. Even newer is the American Medical Joggers Association where first-hand jogging experience is the rule with its members. Doctors learn from their own experience and apply this information to their patients. Some even choose to run with their patients as part of the diagnostic process. Although he is not a runner, Dr. Schuster is considered a pioneer in the sports medicine field. His office in College Point, Queens, New York, is a mecca for runners from all over the country who seek professional help and advice.

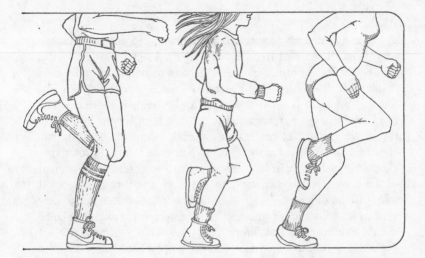

One of the more revolutionary adaptations in athletic diagnosis was generated by Dr. George Sheehan, a New Jersey cardiologist, runner, and pedophile. Many a major athlete has been benched due to knee injuries that may mean surgery and possibly the end of a blossoming career, but Dr. Sheehan, as a runner, noticed that his own injuries, ranging from the top to the bottom of his legs, could often be comfortably resolved by a podiatrist. That treating the foot affected the well-being of the structure above was a simple enough premise, but not one widely recognized before Dr. Sheehan's findings. In fact, those suffering from "runner's knee" (chondromalacia, or softening of the knee cartilage) were generally advised to rest, rely on medication for relief, and practice quadriceps (thigh-muscle) exercises before a decision on surgery could be made. Since doctors have always preferred to use "standard" procedures, this had been the acceptable course of action. But Dr. Sheehan suspected an alternative course. As he wrote about his findings: "This [runner's knee] is a structural—almost architectural—problem; not a medical one."

After treating runners and tennis players with all manner of leg complaints, Dr. Sheehan grew convinced that "we should look first to the feet as the source of trouble." Even the smallest foot disorder will disturb foot and leg alignment and engender leg injury. With the current trend toward vigorous activity and physical fitness, chances of injury increases. Excess activity used to be held responsible for athletically generated injuries and pain, but Dr. Sheehan's insight pointed at a structurally weak foot—which may not have been easily recognized had it not been for the stress factor. A weak foot just can't stand up under the additional athletic strain and weak muscles will exhibit their true colors. If you experience hip or back pain in running, look to your feet. Realignment of the body through conscientious foot care and proper shoes will make all the difference. And with the help of sports medicine, preventive conditioning combined with improved muscle balance should minimize the possibility of any new injury. If you are just beginning a running program, consult a sports medical clinic for professional advice. Once the various muscle groups in the body are balanced, the athlete should be able to perform free of pain and to his or her greatest physical ability.

Sports medicine minimizes the former emphasis on cortisone injections and other such medications as antidotes to foot pain. Instead, the doctor's two primary concerns are strengthening the patient's muscles and treating feet biomechanically. Since a runner's training repeats one set of actions, this means that one main axis of muscles is being used over and over again. As a result, muscle flexibility is assured in the muscles that are exercised, while those not called upon may be fading fast. Complementary exercises will balance the runner's total muscle development and permit him or her to avoid localized strain. One of the beneficial aspects of running is developing in the runner an awareness of the body as a unity—of learning how its different components function together.

After a runner's leg muscles have been performing to the fullest for a while, the runner's foot balance should be examined by a doctor. Often a foot support is recommended to bring the foot to its "ideal" position. This support—an orthosis, or orthotica support, more commonly known as an "orthotic"—theoretically adjusts the foot to a "neutral" position. However, since no one has the perfect foot, adjustment is relative—the foot's position is therefore improved to a point that will not create discomfort. It would be "unrealistic" to seek perfection, Dr. Schuster feels. We tend to think of the body as perfectly vertical when we stand, walk, or run, but our heritage is less than perfect. We may think of the knee and ankle simply as hinges, but the fact is that those joints have built-in components which absorb whatever misalignment might be present.

As eyeglasses are to eyes, orthotics are to feet—they don't correct them; they correct their functioning, to wit, your gait. By putting an orthotic in your shoe, you bring the ground up to meet your foot and prevent the longitudinal arch from flattening and your foot from rolling inward. If an orthotic is made for running shoes, it can be transferred to street shoes, but not vice versa. Casts of feet are made by a podiatrist, and then orthotics are molded from them, from fiberglass, rubber, plastic polymers, or cork. Depending upon the required adjustment, the orthotic may be rigid, flexible, or somewhere in between. For shock absorption, a pillow-type orthotic is used—with soft plastic sponge to soften the impact. Dr. Schuster estimates that this sort of orthotic is more often prescribed to women and older men who may have naturally larger joint ranges and more soft tissue which might require extra protection while running.

The key to relief for the runner's discomfort is to locate the foot imbalance. One leg may be ¼ inch longer than the other. This may not be detectable in walking, but running may make it obvious. In fact, Dr. Schuster says that since more than half his patients show a longer left leg, their symptoms manifest on the right side first. Pounding the ground with four times your body weight will tend to make the longer side rather sore—which a little "lift" in your shoe could easily solve.

Orthotics have enjoyed such great popularity that many runners who don't require them medically ask for them anyway. But unless you need them, they will not improve your performance. A clue to whether your feet are good candidates for them is to check delayed symptoms after a week's running. Do your knees ache? The knee is the number-one site of running disorders, in Dr. Schuster's opinion. This is where orthotics come in handy. Problems usually manifest themselves first in the knee, then down the leg, and finally in the foot itself. When you reach four miles in a ten-mile run, do your symptoms begin? Pain at this point could in-

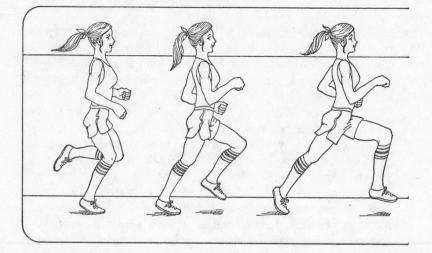

dicate a foot imbalance. More harmful is the "level of anesthesia" that some runners experience after a certain mileage; at this point pain may not register and injuries will more easily occur.

If you notice certain weaknesses in your feet that have not begun to disturb you yet, it may be best not to take any preventive measures. Sometimes the body adapts if left to its own devices, whereas tampering with the latent problem may stir up a hornet's nest. Only if the body is suffering from imbalance will orthotics be of help. As long as the symptom does not develop—keep your fingers crossed and run along.

Dr. Schuster even points out that professional runners have sometimes used orthotics to their detriment; the body may learn to adapt better without outside help. For this reason, Dr. Schuster prescribes orthotics for only two of every five runners who request them—and even then he often suggests that they only be worn for running, since basically his are designed for more comfortable running and minimal fatigue. With proper care, they should last for years with an occasional re-covering.

Sometimes your running shoe may aggravate an existing imbalance in your foot. If you suffer leg discomfort, inspect all possible culprits. Since a running foot is the most variable of all (20 per cent wider and generally more elongated than the average

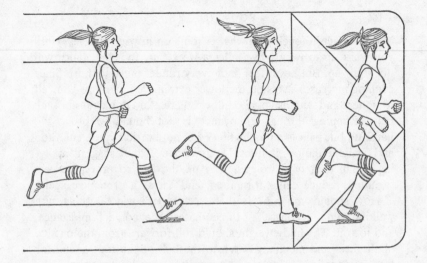

foot), latent problems are apt to manifest themselves. You may
not be wearing the right shoe. With repeated motion you can also
aggravate any irritation on your feet. Store-bought insoles may adjust the position of your feet to a more comfortable level.

Orthotics are actually far from new. In Europe, the first known
orthotic appeared in the 1750s, as an extra piece of inner soling
with protective cut-out areas and stuffing under the arch. Later, in
the nineteenth century, the Germans constructed orthotics of steel
and silver to support structurally delicate feet. Leather soon became the standard material, and now we have a neverending range
of modern synthetic materials to choose from as well.

The key to healthy running feet is preventive medicine—
especially since an estimated 35 to 60 per cent of all runners sport
weak feet. Running specialists Dr. Louis Galli and Dr. Josef Geldwert stress suppleness and strength of all muscles in order to
maintain a happy foot. Warm-up and cool-down exercises are in-
dispensable to ensure cooperation among all muscle groups. A
good warm-up may mean sidestepping muscle pulls and knee and
ankle injuries. After all, running is a sport and should be enjoyed
without painful aftereffects. When you are just beginning, the doctors recommend running for time rather than distance. Try running for ten or fifteen minutes and then walk. Don't push yourself,

but try to get in touch with what is going on in your muscles. Until you work up to twenty-five miles a week, any foot imbalance will not show up. But never fear—not every runner must get hurt. Since running increases stress on the lower extremities, sensitize yourself to understand what is going on down there. And don't run through pain. Running through annoyance is not bound to prove too harmful, but pain is an indication of a more serious problem. Stop and evaluate the possibilities. Dr. Jonathan Zizmor suggests applying a thin coat of petroleum jelly on the feet to prevent excess sweating, reduce callus formation, and act as a protective agent.

How should you run? Is there a "proper" way? Just as with walking, running consists of three phases: heel contact, midstance, and toe off. The body weight should roll forward from the outside of the heel and metatarsal arch to the ball of the foot, rising for toe off. Toes ideally should point straight ahead. There should be a bit of a "rocking" motion sandwiched between heel contact and take off. Unlike the movement in walking, there is a phase in running in which both feet are off the ground. In the case of the long-distance runner or jogger, foot strike should be as light and silent as humanly possible. Beware of any "slapping" as you put your feet down; this may be a sign of flatfeet.

If a runner has an unstable heel, Morton's foot or flattening of the longitudinal arches, future complications are predictable. Some unstable heels turn into "jogger's ankle" which generally manifests itself as pain on the outside of the ankle. This will occur in a foot that rolls outward and naturally leans on the ankle to an excessive degree. When you're exerting six times your body weight at every curve you run, ligaments in the ankle area may succumb to injury. Once the position of the foot is adjusted, peace may be restored.

The Grecian foot with its longer second toe attracts heel spurs and shin splints in runners. When the muscles and tendons of the forefoot are overworked, shin splints develop. These painful swellings appear on the muscles of the front of the lower leg. Beginners are prone to this inconvenience because of the new demands of running on their legs; any drastic change in training may have similar results with the more seasoned runner. Running on your toes or at a forward tilt may be the culprit, but style is not all. In beginners, the muscles may not have been prepared for this rigorous activity and are letting you know. Proper exercises as well as shoe inserts (supports or anterior crests behind the ball of the foot) may help avert this problem. But once shin splints make themselves known, rest and elevate your legs. Ice massages will often provide instant relief. Running backward may help strengthen unused muscles.

Morton's neuroma—the inflammation of the nerve sheath—is another occupational hazard of the foot type characterized by the longer second toe. This usually afflicts the third interspace and makes itself known by sharp pains. Tight footgear or leaning on the toes (as is the dancer's predisposition) have been held accountable here. Rubbing the area will provide minor relief and may produce a "clicking" sensation—attesting to the injury. Excision of the nerve is the most expeditious treatment, although orthotics or other supports may be used as more conservative measures.

A runner's lack of foot arches may be responsible for any of the aforementioned problems, while heel imbalance tends to produce tendinitis in the runner's knee area. If you sense instability in your heel, cut heel lifts or arch cookies out of felt and insert them in your shoe for greater comfort.

Achilles tendinitis rates as one of the most frequent running ailments; it accounts for about 20 per cent of runners' injuries. This tendon inflammation produces a sharp pain which extends from the underside of the heel to the middle of the calf muscle. The pain is worst in the morning and wanes with the day. Running tightens leg and foot muscles which may pull on the Achilles tendon and cause it to swell. Each time the tendon lifts the body weight (about 1,500 times per mile), it grows more irritated. And damage is compounded with each hard run. Once the tendon heals, it shortens and is even more vulnerable to future injury.

The inward roll of the foot also encourages Achilles tendinitis. With your foot at this angle, the Achilles tendon fibers will eventually twist. Check your running shoes by examining the heel; if the outside part in the back is more worn than the rest of the sole, your foot is leaning inward. A low longitudinal arch would also indicate this foot weakness. Until the Achilles tendon heals complete abstinence from running is imperative; swimming or bicycle riding will have to suffice for the time being. Once it recovers, stretching exercises and a limited running program can be resumed.

Doctors in Vancouver, British Columbia, have done research which leads them to believe that Achilles tendinitis is related to gout and can be similarly controlled. Dr. Richard Schuster reads this problem as evidence that man has developed beyond the point of leaning the heel on the ground. After all, he theorizes, we are just recently out of the trees. Look at our gorilla relatives: they all rely on their toes for mobility. Although we are by far the best bipedal walkers, we are not the fastest by any means. Coming up on our toes, we seem to move more efficiently. Watch little babies learning to walk: they lean on their toes. That explains why both men and women like shoes with heels, Schuster remarks. It feels better. Young men bounce down the street, John Travolta-style, at a fast pace, comfortable with this springy gait. "We are past the level foot stage," Dr. Schuster asserts. And without a heel to lean on, Achilles tendinitis will appear. Which explains the new heel lifts on running shoes. Dr. Schuster feels they could rise to a full inch without harming their tenants in the least. And if calf muscles shorten as a result of heel-wearing, they can be stretched out with simple exercises.

Sometimes muscles pull very hard on a bone and produce fractures. Microtraumas from running may pull the muscle away from the heel bone until pain turns on a red alert, and if the pain is ignored, it may mean a displaced bone later. Reduced mileage may be preferable to complete rest as a treatment. An unstable heel or weak longitudinal arch may be at fault here, but with a full-foot orthotic, a complete running program can soon be resumed.

Of all sports studied by experts, ice hockey alone emerges as relatively free of injuries to the feet. Dr. Schuster ascribes this phenomenon to the lacing ritual of the hockey player; by carefully tying the boot, he creates a perfectly rigid support to stabilize the foot.

Of course, the shoes you wear while running may mean the difference between happy or painful running. In 1978, 40 per cent of all shoes bought by men fell into the running-type category.

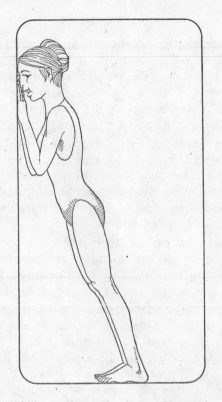

Achilles tendon and calf muscle stretch.

With the obvious rise of interest in running shoes among men and women, it would be wise to bone up on how to evaluate their merits. Of the 175 models produced by over twenty manufacturers —ranging from $20 on up—how do you find the right pair for you?

Podiatrists Galli and Geldwert recommend a hydraulic shoe as ideal since it varies with surface, mileage, pace, and foot structure. "Ideal," however, is a relative term and the shoe must suit your feet. Your age, sex, and type of running will contribute to your decision. With the new sneaker widths, you can look for better fit. If you can bounce around the store before committing yourself, that would be the best situation.

When shopping for running shoes, use this checklist:

■ Is the heel at least ¾ inch higher than the sole? This is important for shock absorption and calf-muscle protection. Pose the
shoes on a table and check that the heels are not leaning in any direction. Cushioning in the heel is particularly important, to prevent pains which may reach up to the lower back.

■ Is the sole two- or three-ply? There should be at least two or
three layers of rubber material, preferably two rigid layers sand-
wiching a spongy middle. Unless you intend to run hills—for which
the "waffle" sole is best suited—crepe rubber soles will give you a
good run for your money. And soles can be easily touched up with
several available commercial products. But don't overdo it—you
don't want to change sole thickness.

■ Does the shoe flex easily? This is a sign of a good shock absorber. Hold the toe and heel in both hands and bend to test.

■ Is there enough room for your feet and cotton socks in the
metatarsal areas? The widest part of your foot should correspond
to the widest part of your shoe. Free toe movement is essential. A
½ inch between your big toe and the shoe toe end should allow
sufficient room and prevent black toenails or blood blisters from
forming. "Jogger's toe" (generally, a simple nail discoloration)
can often be "cured" by switching to a running shoe with a roomier toe area. Tight shoes may also produce a "tingling" sensation
due to the cramped situation of the nerves, but in loose shoes,
friction will of course create blisters. Thick socks would seem to
be the natural defense, but if not, larger blisters should be lanced
with a sterilized needle. Once drained, an antiseptic should be
applied and the blisters covered with an adhesive strip. Dr. Murray Weisenfeld suggests wrapping lamb's wool around blisters to
protect the wound. It is important to treat the blisters before they
interfere with your stride by creating an unnatural imbalance.

"Running is here to stay," affirms Dr. Schuster. All evidence
seems to corroborate this statement. Somehow the euphoria following a good run is good enough inspiration to keep people on
this track. And, as the learned doctor notes, running time allows
people to function in an area of exquisite isolation. Many writers
even attach tape recorders around their necks in order to maxi-
mize on their running time.

Sometimes the heady experience of running with the wind seems to clear away mental cobwebs, tensions, and anxieties; it may even become a problem-solving process. A rhythmic type of meditation may arise as the breathing pattern sets the pace and inward-directed energy connects mind with body. But no matter how you do it or what you do it for, your feet are responsible for carrying you ever onward and deserve just reward for this invaluable service.

# FOOT
# IN THE DOOR

## On the Job

"The shoes that women wear at work have a greater effect on comfort, safety, and efficiency than any other item of clothing," the Women's Bureau of the U. S. Department of Labor reports. And foot ailments account for a high percentage of absenteeism—by no means exclusive to women. Ironically, even though machines have taken over much of the physical labor that used to burden us, foot troubles seem to limit us more than ever before.

Foot fatigue is one of the great facts of life that many people learn to accept. Often our feet can't possibly drag us through an evening's activity after a long day at work. (Everyone knows that liberating feeling once you've kicked off your shoes after you've gotten home from work. Finally you can relax and let your feet stretch out happily outside of their jailer-shoes.) And if you can't make it home soon enough, you'll join in on that age-old chorus: "My feet are killing me!" Yes, they're probably killing your social life, too. And worse, when your feet hurt, you seem to hurt all over.

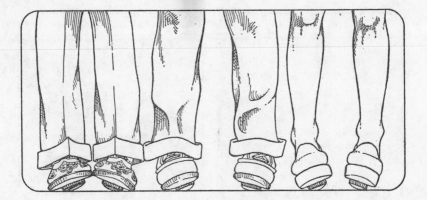

Foot strain is an occupational hazard for people who stand or walk for prolonged periods—salespeople, waiters, waitresses, police, beauticians, and lab technicians, among others. A job which requires long hours in the same position—such as that of an elevator operator—is most demanding on the muscles. The wear and tear of daily life takes its toll with time and you learn that prolonged stress is hard to endure. Standing is a greater strain on the lower extremities than walking since it exerts constant pressure upon the same muscle groups. In addition, you bear down more on the dominant side. Check your soles for the one that shows more wear: if you are right-handed, it should register on the right sole. This natural preference, compounded with latent foot irregularities, can develop into chronic conditions and then affect job performance. The feet feel tired, achy in the arch. The ligaments are working overtime too and they will let you know. Soon your mind is flashing one thought: I want to get off my feet! How can this be avoided? Or can it?

Of course, standing is tiring by definition. Everyone knows that. Even when you stop to chat with a neighbor in the street, you can feel yourself shifting from foot to foot. Concrete pavements are simply not designed with foot comfort as a priority.

If you depend on your feet for your bread and butter, professional care is more important than ever. A podiatrist may be a lifesaver. An ounce of prevention in this case can mean sidestep-

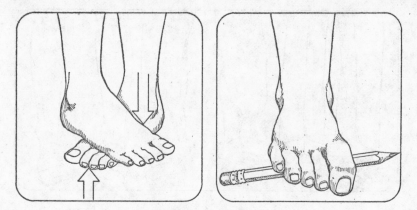

"Foot Press" Exercises

ping needless foot misery. Biomechanical adjustment can mean the difference between wearing a smile or a frown. And if you weren't aware of foot imbalances before, standing at length should serve to raise your consciousness.

Feet may not have been originally meant for weight bearing, but that is now one of their primary functions. And just because you are on your feet all day does not mean they have to hurt any more than your hands do after a hard day's work.

Good standing posture may be a step in the right direction. Pointing one foot straight ahead, pose the other behind it at a 45-degree angle. Lean most of your weight on the ball of the rear foot. Or—for a change of pace—roll onto the outer borders of your feet when they are parallel. This should make upright posture easier to bear by strengthening your arches.

Each occupation attracts a different affliction. For example, a mile of walking will subject your dogs to about 80 tons of weight. A police officer on a beat will find strolling about a trying experience. However, standing in place may develop calcaneal bursitis, more commonly called "policeman's heel." Mailmen and waiters are also vulnerable to this condition. The best preventive measure here is to pad the heels of the shoes for maximum protection. And if the condition flares up, apply heat for relief.

"Waiter's toe" describes the inflammation that arises from kicking a swinging door day after day and catching it with the same

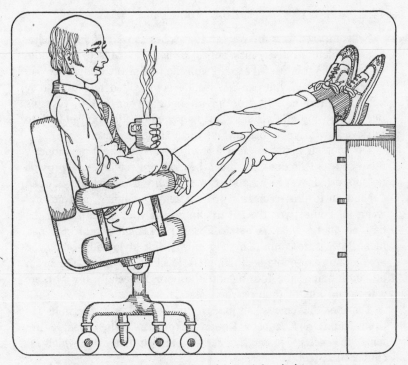

Getting off your feet during the workday is important.

toe. This display of coordination may mean an ingrown toenail later. In fact, repeated small injuries on the job may mean long-term pain and a shortened temper. Stress fractures are aggravated with each motion repeated—a painter who climbs off a ladder, a deliveryman who jumps off a truck in the same way everyday. Sometimes the repercussions of a heavy object dropped on that intrusive little foot may not show up until years later. Since the accumulated impact of imperceptible injuries are out of our range of control, we should learn to sharpen our awareness when we can. If you work with chemicals, special safety shoes should be worn.

If you work in a moist area, beware of insidious fungi. Bartenders and greenhouse and laundry workers should be especially careful. Wear natural-fiber hosiery to absorb perspiration more effectively. Or wear two pairs, wool over cotton, and change them regularly to give your feet a chance to breathe.

Sedentary workers are prey to foot aches as well as anyone else, and complete inactivity may be just as harmful. Muscle tone fades and soon the foot can't keep up with the rest of the body. Take off your shoes when you can and rotate your wilted feet until they come back to life. Do a "foot press" right at your desk by pressing one foot on top of the other. Drop a pencil on the floor and try to retrieve it with your toes to give them some exercise.

Do yourself and your feet a favor by always wearing properly fitted shoes. This does not mean beat-up old scuffies that provide no support. Invest in a good pair of quality shoes which you can depend on to protect against toe stubbing, pounding, and general wear. Of course, you'll want to slip out of your shoes during the day, no matter what. A barefoot coffee break might not be a bad idea. But ensure comfort by choosing a shoe style with roomy toe area and a reasonable heel. Ripple-sole shoes may also ease strain by "cushioning" the foot against the floor, especially for workers who spend lots of time on their feet.

Tension—the enemy of modern man—is also responsible for tired feet. Dr. Elizabeth Roberts explains, "When people are tense, they often become fatigued and this starts a cycle which includes tired feet."

Getting off your feet periodically is also important to good foot maintenance. Occasionally raise your feet above the level of your heart to allow the blood to return upward. Resting at regular intervals during the day should ward off the shuffling effect of foot strain.

Now that machines have taken over much of the physical labor that used to burden our feet, it's about time we took a giant step in foot care rather than reduce our activities.

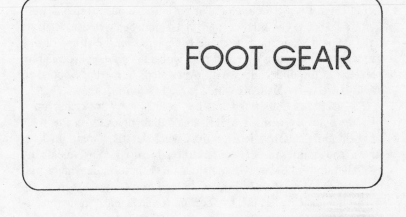

# FOOT GEAR

*"Old friends are best. King James used to call for his old shoes; they were easiest for his feet."*

JOHN SELDEN, 1689

## Stepping Back in Time

Ten thousand years ago or so, man solely relied on his feet for survival. Footgear was a means of protection against the unpredictable elements. And although no shoes that old have yet been unearthed, leather-working tools survive to attest the existence of prehistoric cobblers. As the ice age thawed, agriculture gave rise to new materials and soon sandals woven of leather or grass became the rage. Archaeological evidence shows that everyone was wearing the sandal style fashioned from local materials, from Egyptian papyrus to Arizona yucca. Desert climates required protection from the hot sands against the soles. Soon sandals became more fashionable than functional. Egyptians featured papyrus or leather—although barefooting was equally à la mode.

According to historical consensus, fashion was reserved for the ruling class. By the time King Tut got into sandals, fashions were quite advanced: his sandals were dyed and bejeweled as well as hand painted. A gentle Nile scene is depicted on the straps of one sandal. The king also owned a pair with man's animalistic nature painted on the undersides. With every step, he perhaps hoped to crush these nasty instincts with his mighty foot.

The Hebrews elaborated on the "sole power" look, but on a happier note. By wearing a portrait of their beloved on the soles of their footgear, they left imprints wherever they went. In later times, the courtesans of Alexandria advertised their talents by spelling out "Follow me" in the studs on their soles, leaving a trail of enticing footsteps. Today, some children's sneakers pick up where the ancients left off, by sporting traffic signals on the undersides.

Buffalo-hide sandals known to us today are easily recognizable relatives to their ancestors: flat soles attached to the foot by a single strap over the instep and another over the big toe. The forerunner of the "exercise" sandal was a thick wooden knob held firmly onto the sole by the first and second toes.

Thong-type sandals date back over the centuries to the ancient Chinese. Every culture seems to have worn a variation of this style, from the Japanese with their straw *zori* with the velvet thong to the Greeks with their version which was attached to the foot by a strap above the ankle.

Barefoot was the rule, according to Homer, whose heroes only donned shoes to travel or enter combat. In fact, early Greeks regarded bare feet more highly than shod feet, which were unable to commune directly with the earth. Robert Graves, the author and classicist, theorizes that Greek warriors only required a left shoe to protect the shield side. The left foot was also used to kick the enemy in the groin during the heat of battle. As a result, the left foot developed a bad reputation and—unless an insult was intended—was never extended before the right foot when entering someone's home. It was not until the Hellenistic period (323–31 B.C.) that bare feet were relegated to slaves only. Shoes then began to assume social significance. The Greek biographer Plutarch wrote: "Bare feet, a sign of a slave's degradation."

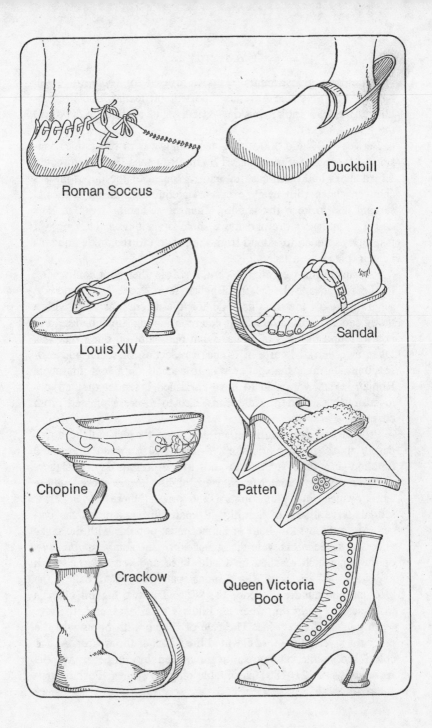

Roman Soccus

Duckbill

Louis XIV

Sandal

Chopine

Patten

Crackow

Queen Victoria Boot

In colder regions, animal skins were used for foot protection. Around 1500 B.C. the Assyrians sported soft leather boots resembling American Indian buskins—laced boots reaching halfway to the knee.

Between 500 and 300 B.C., shoemaking was in full stride, considered more an art than a craft by the Romans. Those who could afford shoes had them custom-made. Women of the upper classes changed shoes with every excuse—sometimes requiring a special servant just to keep the possible changes at hand. Greek sandals began to appear more and more shoelike: a *lingula* (tongue) of leather was added to extend from the toes up to the ankle and was held in place by a lace.

Romans began wearing a *soccus,* a soft leather boot conforming to the foot shape—hence the English term "sock." Designed to separate the big toe from its neighbor, the *soccus* was worn with a thong sandal. This style is still common among the Japanese and is also found in parts of India. What one wore on one's feet was taken as a mark of caste in Rome, a reflection of social and professional stature; what better way to accentuate a toga or tunic? Roman lovers were said to have cherished a sandal of their beloved much as modern Americans used to revere a pressed prom corsage.

Prominent Roman artists then got in on the act and began to design shoes, forcing prices up. Roman fashion soon preempted function—in a takeover that extends to the present day. Designers drew up styles to match each walk of life. *Baxea* were humbly worn by peasants, philosophers, and priests; these woven straw sandals were a sign of humility. Roman citizens sported the *calceus,* an outdoor, low boot of leather most popular with the man-about-town. Senators were distinguished by the somber *cothurnus,* or buskin, which reached up to the knee and was adorned with a golden "C" to signify a Roman patrician (also called the "Roman one hundred," hence the "C"). The two highest officials wore scarlet *cothurni,* whereas Julius Caesar was said to have worn golden soles on his. The rule of thumb with boots was the taller they were, the more elevated the status of the wearer. As for color, red, white, and green were named by Emperor Marcus Aurelius (A.D. 121–180) as suitable only to women. Fashion dictated that white was most suitable for women's shoes, closely followed by yellow and green; Roman brides wore yellow shoes with the white tunics and flame-colored veils. Red was traditionally reserved for the ruling noblemen until Marcus Aurelius benevolently legalized it for women—although not for the common man.

Eventually, the shoe industry got on its feet. Tanners and cobblers organized guilds; armies put in large orders and soon import-export activity was underway. St. Crispin—a shoemaker by trade—preached during the day and worked by night, making shoes to give the poor. His generosity prompted others to question his motives. Were heavenly or satanic forces behind his actions? When Crispin refused to confirm any of their suspicions and withheld information, he was martyred—in A.D. 287. And now he is known as the patron saint of shoemakers everywhere.

An exciting innovation was introduced in the thirteenth century, soon after the Crusades, when Eastern fashions finally hit the West. In the Orient, pointy-toed footwear was assumed to strip witches of supernatural powers. This irresistible attraction was responsible for the immediate popularity of this style among both men and women. In England, this shoe became known as the "crackow" and in France as the *poulaine*. The points of the shoe grew ever longer—sometimes requiring whalebones to keep the leather from flopping about. Intricate designs were brightly inlaid in cloth and velvet. Geoffrey Chaucer describes crackows in *The Miller's Tale* (c. 1387). Despite the ever-growing point, the style kept in step, peaking around 1460 when it extended as far as 12 inches beyond the end of the foot. At this length, it was tied to the knee and came to be regarded as a sign of great wealth.

In 1305 Edward I of England came up with the concept of shoe sizes. Using barleycorns as the standard of measure, thirty-nine placed in a row were considered to represent the longest "normal" foot possible; that size was named "13" and smaller sizes were calculated from there, each separated by one barleycorn (about ⅓ inch). This made it easier for a wealthy man to order shoes from the cobbler. And cobblers could work faster with the invention of the iron needle, a shoemaking innovation.

In the 1400s, "pattens"—sandals worn over shoes in the protective manner of galoshes—came into vogue; they could be worn over *poulaines* to keep them out of the mud. Occasionally, pattens had platform soles of iron, wood, or cork. This style was so effective that it lasted well into the 1800s. Actually, platform shoes had already appeared in the third century B.C. on the Greek stage. Actors felt that the few extra inches contributed to their stage presence. Aeschylus required thick cork soles to convey this larger-than-life image. In 1926 Emperor Hirohito of Japan emulated this notion by climbing on 12-inch *geta* (platforms) as a majestic gesture for his coronation.

In reaction to the long reign of pointy shoes, wide shoes drew attention during the reign of Francis I of France (1494–1547). Shoes with the "duckbill"-look also featured sumptuous linings. The wider the toe, the more dignified the status of its wearer. This style is often attributed to Henry VIII of England, Francis I's contemporary, who was said to have designed it to accommodate his painfully sensitive gout-stricken feet. Soon the style caught on among his courtiers. In fact, a ponderous gait—inevitable with this clumsy style—came to be considered a sign of the upper classes. Because of the ever-widening toe box, Queen Mary I (1516–58) was later forced to put her foot down and limit the fashion to 6 inches across.

Heels are attributed to the inventive Catherine de Médicis (1519–89), Queen of France. They were originally simply lifts attached to flat slippers, without any consideration for the arch. In England, highwaymen cleverly devised removable heels to conceal small booty such as jewelry. Until the French Revolution, heels inspired the imagination of many an artist and craftsman. Shapes varied to the most whimsical—even *bons mots* were stitched into their sides. Frivolity was the rule of foot.

The heel craze grew with the introduction of "chopines"—platform shoes. Although this style had long enjoyed popularity in the East, it only attracted moderate interest in the West until the sixteenth century. The style was introduced by way of Turkish harems and Venice. Interest shifted from the front of the foot to the rear as platforms reached new heights of up to 2 feet. Even Hamlet ventured a fashion-conscious remark: "By 'r lady, your ladyship is nearer to heaven than when I saw you last, by the altitude of a chopine." Elevated to new heights, women sometimes found it easier to walk when flanked by two servants. The attraction seemed to be found in this confirmation of female fragility and dependence. Meanwhile the Church exulted as dancing was abandoned for the less pleasurable activity of tottering about on stiltlike shoes.

Men, too, indulged their pedal fantasies; boots rose to new heights, now adorned with heels and spurs. Rosettes, buckles, and bows appeared. French King Louis XIV (1638–1715), a diminutive head of state, was especially partial to heels and, in fact, the "Louis heel" is named after him. He was very proud of a pair of red high heels sporting bows which reached 8 inches on either side of the knot, complete with two smaller bows at each end.

Buckles were making their debut at this time on the famed feet of Samuel Pepys (1633–1703), the English diarist. This look was adopted by the early American colonists who set up shop in Salem, Massachusetts. Previously shoes had been fastened with "latchets," or leather thongs. The appearance of buckles changed the look of the shoe significantly.

At the time of the French Revolution in 1789, heels were banished. Women padded about in soft, flat slippers. Simple pumps, hitherto worn only by footmen, were now commonly worn by all male citizens. This new movement put the 20,000 English buckle makers of Birmingham out of business. Not even the Prince of Wales could persuade his people to wear last year's styles.

Patent leather quietly appeared on the scene in the early nineteenth century, manufactured in Paris and in Newark, New Jersey, but capricious footwear for women was strictly taboo in Victorian times. Long skirts kept shoes out of sight and prevented any undue interest. For men, gaiters eased the transition from boots to shoes. Originally used in boots, these pieces of felt or leather buttoned around the leg at the sides of the boot, dispensing with fasteners altogether. Later on, gaiters became a separate entity worn over the shoe.

The Americans meanwhile were getting on their feet as an industrial force; shoe manufacturing was on the rise as exports of footwear to Europe increased and "ready-made" shoes became available in all sizes and in right–left configurations. By 1820 the United States was a mass producer of footwear for the world. What had started out as a constructive way for people to pass the time when not farming, became a prosperous industry. Farming families used to tan leather; then traveling cobblers would pass through to make the family shoes.

In terms of style, Americans are responsible for three distinct shoe fashions: the Indian moccasin, the cowboy boot, and· the good old sneaker. The sneaker—originally a "croquet sandal"— first appeared in *The Peck and Snyder Sporting Goods Catalog* in the 1860s. By 1897 the mail-order firm of Sears, Roebuck & Company was widely advertising the shoes at 60 cents a pair. The term "sneaker" crept into newspaper ads sometime in the 1870s, never to be deposed, despite specialization into "tennis shoes," "running shoes," and "squash shoes."

Before they appeared in the U.S., primitive versions of sneakers had been long worn in the Amazon basin. Brazilian Indians fashioned these sturdy shoes by stepping into the sap of rubber trees and then allowing it to dry on their feet, for perfect fit. But it was Charles Goodyear's rubber vulcanization process that made sneakers widely available in the late nineteenth century—although he did not live to witness their vast popularity.

Shoes came to be regarded as accessories in the twentieth century, designed to enhance one's wardrobe without much regard to function. And today, as specialty shoes for every occasion vie for the limelight—from opera pumps to hiking boots—attention on our taken-for-granted feet increases. Footwear is an expression of personality; even the most conservative businessman can make a subtle statement with his choice of shoes. Surprising footwear can be a telling clue; Woody Allen has been snapped with First Lady Betty Ford and Martha Graham—in tux and sneakers.

The Footwear Council, a spokesman for the footwear industry of America, simplifies the boggling array of shoe styles by arranging them into seven general categories: sandal, mule, moccasin, boot, pump, monk strap, oxford. Everything else is just a variation on one of these standard designs, variations that change seasonally to appease the natural desire to enhance our feet.

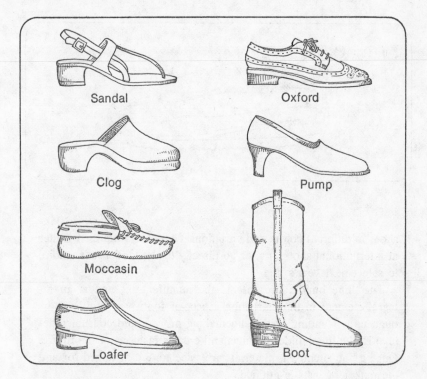

Sandal

Oxford

Clog

Pump

Moccasin

Loafer

Boot

## The Straight and Narrow

For 2,000 years, Italy has greatly influenced shoe fashion, as illustrated by the Italian terms used in the shoe industry. The shoe "modelista" (master designer) carries on an ancient tradition, attracting buyers from all over the world. Fashion sense, creativity, and foresight contribute to the vision; expertise in shoe construction and manufacture are called upon for the creation of the design. When inspiration strikes, the modelista makes a pull-over —a model attached to a wooden block in the shape of a foot. (In America, designers prefer to use sketches.) Using this pull-over as a basis, the modelista creates variations on this theme until a "line" emerges. Each expert usually develops a specialty: sandals, dress shoes, boots. A "line" may consist of one of these types of shoes in different colors and variations. Manufacturers then gather at international shoe fairs, or go directly to the modelista's studio, to select next year's line.

The "line builder" represents the manufacturer and is an integral element in the marketing aspect of footwear. With a thorough understanding of the shoemaking process and consumer demands, the line builder predicts and creates fashions of the future. Once a line is chosen, materials are selected and arranged for and the maker of lasts is notified.

Making a shoe requires ten basic steps, whether it is hand- or machine-made. Eighty different types of machines may be needed in the creation of a single shoe.

1. The first step is constructing the last, the foot-shaped model that simulates the dynamic mass of the foot. It is usually sculpted from wood by hand to ensure correct dimensions. The material for the upper part of the shoe is fitted over the last and the sole is attached afterward. An archaeological expedition in Switzerland unearthed a last made in about 2000 B.C.—giving us an idea as to how early the principles of shoemaking were recognized. Today, shoe factories may house thousands of lasts for every size, width, heel height, and toe design. Duplicate lasts have been used since 1961 to help shoe production, even upstaging their wooden forefathers in many cases. The tradition is preserved in the expression "on the wood," to mean the fitting process of the upper part of the shoe.

2. Now the pattern maker transfers the original sketches in crayon onto the last itself. Corresponding shapes of paper are then pinned onto the last. Once the desired contours are attained, the paper model becomes the pattern for the shoe-to-be.

3. Paper cut-outs are replaced by leather counterparts which must be 100 per cent accurate. The upper is pieced together and lined, if necessary. (The upper consists of the various components of the shoe that protect the top of the foot.) Once the upper is ready, it is pulled over the last and tacked down for the sole and heel. It is now called a "trial," since it is a sample shoe (generally size 6B) which will be modified according to the line builder's wishes.

4. When a line is finally selected, the materials are cut in mass quantity to fill orders. Special cutting machines—even laser beams—are used to cut the leather into different sizes.

5. Detail work on the shoes follows: buttonholes, stitching or ornamental designing. The components are all attached to build a shoe—the lining, counters (heel reinforcers), and toe boxes (toe reinforcers).

6. Back at the last, the upper is checked again for good shape and design. This process can take up to two days or just the amount of time needed to sole and heel the upper.

7. Preparation of the sole is called "stock fitting" and includes an insole, sock lining, shank, outsole, and heel. Both sock lining and insole are attached to the upper; the toe seam is then cemented down while the sides of the instep are stapled and the heel is tacked down.

8. At this stage, the shoe is taken to the bottoming room where the shank and outsole will be attached to the upper. There are three options in this process, depending on the shoe style: cementing—this applies to from 60 to 70 per cent of soles and is easily recognized by the absence of stitching which makes it more difficult to resole; molding—including the vulcanizing of rubber soles as in sneakers; sewing—à la the moccasin technique.

9. As icing on a cake, the heel is now attached. Often it is outsized and needs to be honed down.

10. Final touches such as a complete polish, removal of the shoe from the last, insole pads insertion, and labelling prepare the shoes for the packing room. Any incidental damage, which can easily occur in the manufacturing process, is remedied here and trim or laces added.

## If the Shoe Fits . . .

*"A healthy foot walks optimally without shoes on a soft surface."*
DR. ELIZABETH ROBERTS

Dr. Bernard Rosenstein, of the Columbia Presbyterian Medical Center in New York, gives us a rule of foot good-humoredly dubbed "Rosenstein's Law": *If a shoe is attractive, it doesn't fit.* "You might as well tie a noose around your neck if you insist on wearing those crazy styles," he adds. To satisfy your own curiosity, place your shoe beside your foot and compare the two. Is there any resemblance in shape? Most feet are roughly triangular, with the base of the triangle running along the top of the toes, whereas some shoes have a reverse triangular shape. So we trap our triangular feet into the reverse configuration and expect to prance about without any discomfort for the rest of our lives. It doesn't take a crystal ball to foresee a fall here.

Custom-made shoes don't always fit, either. Sometimes the impression of the foot may be imperfect and will differ a fraction of an inch from the original—enough to cause irritation. Remember, ⅓ inch represents a complete size difference, as from a size 8B to 9B.

Shoe expert Dr. Malcolm Jacobson of the Bellevue Hospital Center in New York and one of the Jacobson Brothers, makers of orthopedic shoes, does not understand why some of his patients are *not* pulling out their hair in agony. In fact, Dr. Jacobson speculates that almost every adult American woman possesses a pair of abused feet; but as long as their feet don't hurt too much, most women allow their foot problems to go untreated. He estimates of

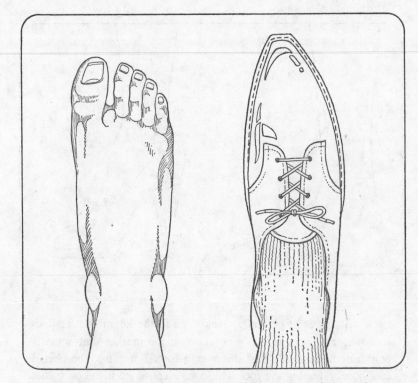

Compare the natural shape of your foot to the
shape of your shoe.

the quarter million pairs of ailing feet he has examined thus far, in
the majority of cases women who have worn atrocious shoes can
get away with it without developing any crippling disabilities. Of
course, this also depends on the pain-tolerance threshold; many
people are willing to sacrifice comfort for style. And these fashion-conscious shoe buyers often prove that even when we put
them through the grinder, we land on our feet.

Dr. Jacobson ascribes many of the foot woes suffered by both
men and women to the fallacy that shoes are mirror images of our
feet. We already have seen that this is not the case—and, to boot,
one foot is always slightly larger than its partner. No one has two
identical feet. As a result, ready-made shoes—necessary evils, per-

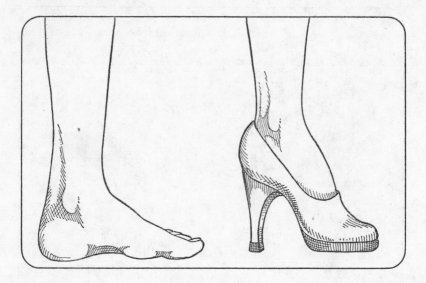

haps—will never fit perfectly, even if we fit the larger foot as doctors suggest. There is really no shoe on the market that actually conforms to the outline of the human foot. For some, the heel·is too loose, releasing the foot with each step. Since the shoe comes off the last by pulling the whole form from the rear, the heel has to be fairly wide. That's why it is virtually impossible for some people to find a snug heel.

The person looking for heel fit then buys smaller, tighter shoes in search of a snug heel that will control foot movement. As a result, toes are often cramped. Cinderella's Prince Charming had it easy compared to the contemporary quest for the perfect shoe. Fitting does not mean heel fitting; when the heel feels firm and in control as the foot's rudder, this does not guarantee a happy forefoot. High-heeled pumps are the worst offenders in this case, causing heel abrasion and the formation of calluses due to friction. Excess tightness in front may coax out latent bunions.

In fact, high heels are most often held responsible for foot problems. "How can you walk in those six-inch heels?" is a frequent query to the fashionably shod. In truth, no one is sure how they hobble from point A to point B—but it seems that style for some must be maintained at any cost. When stiletto heels caught on in the early 1960s, patients asked one podiatrist what he thought of them. "I think they will put all my kids through college," he responded wryly.

Even if you don't feel today the ill effects of staggering about on skinny high heels, you'll be sorry later—when your feet give in to years of abuse. Wearing high heels is not a mistake in itself: wearing them nonstop is. Body weight that should be supported by the entire foot is thrust upon the ball of the foot. Heavy calluses develop at the metatarsal area and toes may jam against the top of the shoe. Faulty balance can lead to sprained ankles and strained backs. Often, high-heeled shoes contain convex soles which cause side-to-side rocking; the leg muscles responsible for body stability are then strained and may hurt. (A short, rigid insole could provide relief.) Sometimes the calf muscles shorten permanently due to constant heel lift, and even houseshoes may have to be heeled for greater comfort.

Platform shoes have challenged heels for the title of "most harmful style to feet" by putting the body in even more precarious situations. With foot flexibility gone, instinct and stumbling alone guide your feet forward. There is no contact with the ground and no toeing off; as a result, there is limited use of intrinsic foot muscles. In addition, perched upon a platform shoe presents an unstable situation, and any false move may mean injury to the ankle.

Boots are equally guilty in crimes against the feet. Dr. Elizabeth Roberts considers them "crazy" for all-day wear, especially for people with circulatory problems. Because of the compression of tight boots, inflammatory conditions are apt to develop. In addition, they are heavy to carry around and should not be worn all day long. If you waterproof them with silicone, they will not be able to breathe and your feet will live in a very moist environment. Don't forget: boots were originally designed for utilitarian purposes and not for style—and that is still an aspect to their function.

Some shoe designers sought to prove that the negative heel—one lower than the toe of the shoe—was the solution to all comfort problems. The roomy toe area was a great attraction for buyers, but the negative heel was not the answer to foot problems. Although heel height is an issue, there is still a considerable difference between no heel and a depression at the heel—which creates new complications in the calf muscles and Achilles tendon. When there is a shortened muscle, tendons may rupture. Shifting body weight is always a serious consideration, certain to involve secondary effects. Wearing a negative heel is equivalent to walking uphill all the time. Only if a doctor wishes to decrease stress on the ball of the foot or if a runner is training for better push-off should this measure be taken.

Another alleged culprit where the lower extremities are concerned is stretch pantyhose. Dr. Jacobson feels that they run a close second to shoes in deforming feet by bunching up at the toes and causing unnatural toe positions. Excess pressure from snug hose may then bring out latent hammertoes. Socks or stockings in exact specific sizes tend to fit better, whereas stretch pantyhose may slip and cramp the toes.

Doctors seem to concur that a lightweight, flexible leather shoe with a lace is the most desirable, since it can be adjusted to personal taste. It's simply an extension of that old stand-by for children, the low, broad-heeled oxford. Unfortunately, styles do not promote this medical advice.

Leather is an important element in good footwear since it is porous; synthetic materials will not ventilate and chances of fungal infection or dermatitis will increase. Good construction is also vital. Often cemented soles will give way while the sewn variety may retain their shapes longer. If you want your shoes to keep their shape, shoe trees can help; newspaper stuffed into the toes of shoes is just as good.

The more fashionable open-toed and -heeled sandals for women are also medically approved footwear. Dr. Roberts swears by hers, which are sensibly low (heels no taller than 1½ inches) and wide enough to give all her toes room to move. And she can perform "face lifts" on sandals to accommodate the shape of a troubled foot just as comfortably as would an orthopedic shoe, and more attractively, as well.

When it comes to a single style that doctors are enthusiastic about, they respond in a loud voice: sneakers. "I love them!" says one. "My kids wear sneakers all the time—except to formal events," reveals another. "On all counts, the sneaker is ideal." Claims another, "Perfect heel height and fit and the washable upper minimize the chance of dermatological infection." And still another: "Sneaker soles are best for shock absorption."

From a style once regarded as sloppy or too informal—even a sign of poverty—the sneaker appears on the feet of numerous celebrities. Woody Allen swears by them; Mick Jagger wore them to his wedding. Andy Warhol says: "They feel like you're wearing pillows."

What is behind the sneaker cult?

Some shoe manufacturers see this change in sneaker status as a sign of a change in life-style. In the 1950s sneakers were solely teenage gear, worn to the hop and elsewhere because of peer pressure. But since the emphasis on physical fitness during President John F. Kennedy's administration, sneakers have enjoyed a boom. Compounded with the new televised specialty sports programs—especially the Olympics—the public has been constantly exposed to this new, attractive, sporty look. When the running look caught on in the late 1960s, that was the clincher. Trend setters saw sneakers as a comfortable way of sidestepping the rigid formalities of yore. Adidas running shoes set the pace for the hundreds of variations to come, ranging from leather to suede to canvas uppers and yet all universally known as "sneakers."

As the consumer grew more sophisticated, manufacturers had to comply by providing different widths in sneakers—hitherto produced in only an average width. New names appeared to describe the new styles and differentiate between functions. Keds—the age-old line recognized by mothers for quality children's sneakers—branched out: Pro-Keds appeared for the older set and Grass-hoppers for women. One distributor of sneakers even cleverly disguised them as sedate business shoes for dog-tired bankers.

But what can you wear when sneakers are taboo and you're looking for comfort? Are orthopedic shoes the solution? Not really, in the opinion of the experts. It all depends on the individual case. Of course, it is imperative to consult a podiatrist to ascertain the right course of action. Molded shoes should certainly be a last resort. Although you should get a custom fit, the main disadvantage to molded shoes is their hefty weight. As a result, a foot wearing them generates more heat and new problems are created. Also, because of the less-than-perfect casts—taken while the foot is at rest, for example—the shoe is often too short. And if the foot impression is taken while standing, the longitudinal arch may flatten out and create other discrepancies. Elongated, flexible feet are bad candidates for this type of shoe, whereas a rigid arthritic foot is best. Be selective since orthopedic shoes are a major investment (between $100 and $350).

It might be more economical to compromise. For example, if you have a bunion, buy wider ordinary shoes. Although it may seem snug about the bunion, this shoe can be stretched to the desired width, while an insole can take up the slack on the other foot.

How can we choose our shoes wisely without sacrificing style? Scientific principles of fit have to be discarded since they don't apply to most of the shoes available on the market. One doctor calls the shoe industry "immoral" for thinking more of the convenience of inventory than of the life in our feet. With so much scientific information on foot function available, why aren't shoes more comfy?

First of all, we must take our genes into account: what problems do we see in our parents' feet? What are our predispositions? Do we want to chance hammertoes by wearing tight, pointy shoes? And, then there are the "hereditary" shopping factors: our parental buying habits. Salespeople are not foot experts and their interests may conflict with those of our feet. Designers only give them styles to work with—not medical answers to foot pain. However, "Man was cruel to his feet long before shoe designers came on the scene," remarks Dr. Roberts.

Avoid pitfalls by protecting yourself as a consumer: as a safeguard, make sure that the money you spend on shoes is refundable and don't be shy about good fit. Wear the shoes at home on a carpeted area or put a sock around the shoe to check for pinching without scuffing the shoe. Ideally, shoes should be bought in midafternoon since feet swell during the course of the day and your shoes should accommodate this. However, this consideration should not affect your shoe shopping too seriously since the swelling is almost imperceptible in most cases. But if you like to be on the safe side, buy shoes during a late lunch hour.

Don't concentrate solely on heel fit in a shoe, since the toe is equally important to gait and foot function—besides being more vulnerable to foot injury. Shoe fitting is an art rather than a science and is based on the shoe seller's highly trained sense of "feel." With the depersonalized service in most stores today, we tend to rush through the shoe buying process without getting fitted.

In fitting shoes, two measuring devices—the Ritz stick and the Brannock metal fitting tray—rule supreme. Don't simply ask for your size: ask to be fitted. And make the salesperson do it while you are standing and for both feet. Your larger foot is usually the left foot, so don't let the salesperson stop with the right. If there is a considerable difference in size between your feet, opt for a larger size and use an inner sole for the smaller foot. But buy for fit rather than size.

To check for good fit experts recommend stepping on top of the shoe with your bare foot. With the shoe flattened out this way, about an inch of leather should extend beyond the tip of your toe. If you're not allowing your toes enough room, this might explain a lot of your foot aches.

Leather or canvas are porous materials and thereby the most congenial materials to wrap around your feet. Shoe soles should preferably be of leather as well, to keep moisture at bay. But we also have to live with rubber—which just might mean using a foot deodorant. There should be no such thing as "breaking in" your shoe—or, more likely, your foot. A small amount of shoe stiffness may be noticeable at first, but it should not cause blisters and require adhesive strips.

Important qualities in a shoe are good shank (instep) curves and properly balanced heel seats. When too low, the shank will irritate the metatarsals and result in foot fatigue. Flat heel seats will hurt the heel, while forward-slanting ones will hurt the forefoot.

As for clogs, opinion is mixed. Of course, the Dutch have been clomping about in them outdoors for centuries, without any apparent problems. Most doctors believe that a rigid wooden sole

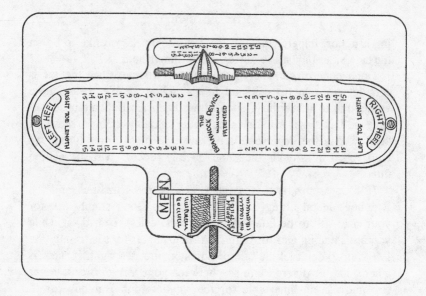

will provide support for a flatfoot. But for those unused to wearing them, false moves may shatter fragile bones or sprain an unsteady ankle—especially in the open-back "Swedish" style.

When walking on city streets, a thick leather sole is desirable for protection, as well as a sensible, broad-based heel. A thick sole need not be stiff; on the contrary, since stiff soles would mean walking awkwardly and instant fatigue. For maximum walking comfort, look for a shoe with a flexible sole at the ball where the foot bends.

Check the shank of the shoe—the bridge between the heel and sole beneath the longitudinal arch—for rigidity. Many shoes, such as loafers, have flexible shanks which may mean arch strain or heel pain if worn frequently. The wedge-heel style, worn by nurses and waitresses, offers more support and is preferable as everyday wear.

Once the foot "moves in"—that is, makes its individualized contour inside the shoe—all should be well. If the heel counter (the stiffener that gives form to the upper part of the back of the shoe) is too stiff at first, "roll" it until it becomes more pliable. Insoles may help keep you on your feet while the leather softens.

Shoe care could extend the lives of your shoes if you make the effort. The key here is maintenance. To keep leather lustrous, it is important to polish with paste or wax, not liquid polish, to restore the natural oils which soon fade. The principle is analogous to skin care: when chapped, apply cream. Leather gets chapped too, and liquid polish will only serve to smother the shoe.

The secret to blending fashion with comfort is to change footgear during the day. As long as you vary heel heights during the day, you will not put undue stress on any one muscle group. Some experts recommend crepe soles as both sensible and stylish.

Although doctors don't like to generalize about shoes, since feet are such variable darlings, an APA poll showed that Clark's Wallabies, Wedgies, and sneakers ranked at the top.

Yet, when it comes down to a question of beauty versus health, most of us—vain creatures—prefer to appear glamorous, even if we must contend with aches and pains. But keeping up with fashion does not have to be incompatible with good foot care. By taking little preventative measures daily, you could be walking on air for a lifetime.

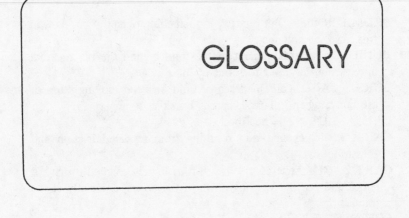

# GLOSSARY

**ACHILLES TENDON.** The tendon which connects the calf muscles to the heel.

**ACUPUNCTURE.** A Chinese form of treatment involving the use of special needles.

**ACUTE INJURY.** A sudden injury.

**ARCH, LONGITUDINAL.** The heel-to-toe arc formation of bones, sustained by muscles and ligaments in each foot.

**ARCH SUPPORT.** A foot appliance which can be built into a shoe or made as a removable device, designed to act as a crutch for shaky arches. Sometimes called a "cookie" due to its uncanny resemblance to that after-school treat.

**ARTHRITIS.** A degenerative joint disease.

**ASTRINGENT.** A substance that controls secretions and causes tissues to contract.

**BALL OF THE FOOT.** The metatarsal area, that is, the fleshy region of the sole behind the toes.

**BIOMECHANICS.** The branch of medical engineering concerned with the dynamics of human motion.

BLISTER.   An irritation that causes fluid to collect under the skin.

BROMIDROSIS.   Put bluntly, foul-smelling perspiration, and, in this case, smelly feet.

BUNION.   An enlargement of the joint behind the big toe that may throw the other toes out of line.

BURSA.   A self-contained sac of fluid between moving parts of the body; when inflamed, causes bursitis.

CALCANEUS.   The heel bone.

CALLUS.   Thickened skin resulting from repeated friction and pressure.

CARTILAGE.   The connective fibrous tissue designed to absorb shock and prevent wearing down of the bones, especially at the joints.

CHIROPODIST.   An old-time foot doctor.

CLUB NAIL.   Deformed thickened nail caused by an injury.

CORN.   A cone-shaped horny formation usually found on the toes as a result of localized pressure or friction.

FALLEN ARCH.   A collapsed longitudinal arch due to weakened ligaments.

FASCIA.   A sheet of internal fibrous tissue encasing parts of the body.

FISSURES.   Cracks often found between the toes or at the heel.

FLATFOOT.   *Acquired:* A collapsed longitudinal arch caused by bad walking habits, overweight, or weak ligaments. *Congenital:* A foot having a flat longitudinal arch from birth.

GAIT.   One's manner of walking.

GOUT.   A form of arthritis generally involving the big toe, caused by a metabolic imbalance (usually an excess of uric acid in the blood).

HALLUX.   The big toe.

HALLUX RIGIDUS.   A joint deformation that limits movements of the big toe.

HALLUX VALGUS.   A condition in which the big toe deviates toward the outside of the foot.

HAMMERTOE.   A contracted or buckled toe, most commonly found in the second toe.

HEEL LIFT. An extra layer of leather in the heel of a shoe, usually no more than ¼ inch thick.

HEMATOMA. A swelling containing blood, often found under the nail after injury.

HYPERHIDROSIS. Excessive sweating.

INGROWN TOENAIL. A nail that pierces the flesh around it due to improper cutting or tight shoes.

INTERMITTENT CLAUDICATION. Pain in the leg muscles after a measured number of steps, caused by a circulatory problem.

LAST. A foot-shaped model used in shoe construction.

MARCH FRACTURE. A bone fracture in the metatarsal group.

MATRIX OF THE NAIL. Area of the toe from which the nail emerges.

METATARSAL AREA. The ball of the foot which contains the five metatarsal, or long, bones. These bones, which are arched, function as levers in pushing body weight forward.

METATARSAL PAD. A protective device inserted in the shoe or attached to the foot to prevent injury to the metatarsal area or to a fallen metatarsal arch.

NAIL BED. The toe area seen through the transparent portion of a nail.

NAIL GROOVE. The border between the side of the nail and the skin.

ONYCHOMYCOSIS. A fungal infection of the nail, recognized by a yellowish discoloration.

ORTHOPEDIST. A doctor specializing in restoring or correcting deformities of the skeletal system.

ORTHOTIC. A shoe insert designed to improve the foot's relationship to the surface underfoot; often used by runners to improve performance.

PHALANGES. Toe bones.

PLANTAR WART. A wart on the sole of the foot.

PODIATRIST. A doctor trained to treat the foot and all its ailments.

PRONATION. The tendency to roll the feet toward each other when standing.

REFLEXOLOGY.   A modern medical technique that allegedly treats all body disorders by applying pressure to specific points on the foot.

SESAMOIDS.   Two small bones lodged in the tendon behind the big toe.

SHIATSU.   A Japanese form of body massage which relies on techniques particularly involving the thumbs and palms.

SHIN SPLINTS.   Muscle injury or inflammation in the front of the leg from overexertion or foot imbalance.

SPICULE.   A needle-shaped particle of bone or nail.

SPRAIN.   Torn ligament fibers.

SPUR.   A projection of bone commonly found at the heel as a result of undue pressure.

STRAIN.   The same thing as a "pull"—the tearing of muscle fibers in a muscle or tendon.

TAILOR'S BUNION.   A bunion on the outside of the fifth toe associated with the old-time tailor's cross-legged position.

TALUS.   The ankle bone.

TENDINITIS.   Inflammation of a tendon.

TENDON.   A fibrous cord that attaches muscles to bones.

ULCER.   A break in tissue leading to further disintegration of tissue.

ULTRASOUND.   A form of therapy using mechanical vibrations.

UPPER.   The upper components of a shoe.

WART.   A benign tumor probably caused by a virus.

# LIST OF SOURCES

## Books

Berkeley Holistic Center. *The Holistic Health Handbook*. Berkeley: Andover, 1978.

Carter, Mildred. *Helping Yourself with Foot Reflexology*. New York: Parker, 1973.

Ewart, Charles. *The Healing Needles*. New York: Keats, 1973.

Fast, Julius. *You and Your Feet*. New York: St. Martin's, 1971.

Galton, Lawrence. *Medical Advances*. New York: Penguin, 1977.

Garten, M. O. *The Natural and Drugless Way for Better Health*. New York: Parker, 1969.

Glover, Bob, and Jack Shepherd. *The Runner's Handbook*. New York: Penguin, 1978.

Graziano, Joseph. *Footsteps to Better Health*. Graziano, 1973.

Hass, Frederick J., M.D., and Edward F. Dolan, Jr. *The Foot Book*. Chicago: Regnery, 1973.

Ingham, Eunice. *Stories the Feet Have Told*. Ingham, 1959.

Irwin, Yukiko. *Shiatsu.* Philadelphia: Lippincott, 1976.

Law, Donald. *A Guide to Alternate Medicine.* New York: Hippocrene, 1974.

Leach, M., ed. *Funk & Wagnall's Standard Dictionary of Folklore, Myth and Legend.* New York: Funk & Wagnall, 1949.

Lust, John. *The Herb Book.* New York: Bantam, 1974.

Mann, Felix. *Acupuncture.* New York: Vintage, 1973.

Mattfeld, Julius. *Variety Music Cavalcade.* Englewood Cliffs, N.J.: Prentice-Hall, 1971.

Radford, E. and M. A. *Encyclopedia of Superstition.* New York: Greenwood, 1969.

Roberts, Elizabeth, D.P.M. *On Your Feet.* New York: Pyramid, 1975.

Rossi, William. *The Sex Life of the Foot and the Shoe.* New York: Ballantine, 1976.

Sheehan, George, M.D. *Dr. Sheehan on Running.* New York: Bantam, 1978.

Stevenson, Burton, ed. *The Home Book of Proverbs.* New York: Macmillan, 1948.

Turner, R. *The Mode in Footwear.* New York: Scribner's, 1948.

Vincent, L. M., M.D. *The Dancer's Book of Health.* Mission: Sheed, Andrews & McMeel, 1978.

Walker, Samuel A. *Sneakers.* New York: Workman, 1977.

Zizmor, Jonathan, M.D. *Dr. Zizmor's Brand-Name Guide to Beauty Aids.* New York: Harper & Row, 1978.

# Pamphlets

*All About Shoes.* New York: Footwear Council, 1979.

*Feet and Their Care.* Chicago: Scholl, Inc., 1978.

*Foot Facts.* Philadelphia: "Penn-Pod" Foot Health Series, University of Pennsylvania, 1955.

Zerinsky, Sidney. *The Swedish Massage Workbook.* New York: Swedish Institute, 1975.

## Articles

Brody, Jane. "Personal Health," New York *Times,* May 10, 1978, and February 14, 1979.

Conniff, James C. G. "Getting on a Good Footing," New York *Times,* April 23, 1978.

Ettlinger, Catherine. "Footnews," *House & Garden,* June 1978.

Hamilton, Dr. William. "Ballet and Your Body," *Dance Magazine,* August/September 1978.

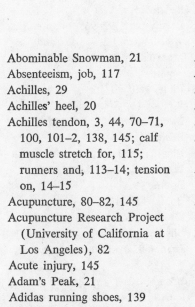

# INDEX

## About the Author

Michelle Arnot received her education at Beloit College and Columbia University. She is a free-lance writer whose health-related articles have appeared in many magazines, including *Esquire, Travel and Leisure,* and *Glamour;* she also constructs crossword puzzles which are syndicated in newspapers throughout the country. Ms. Arnot lives with her husband in New York City where, in her spare time, she is busy running, dancing, and walking. FOOT NOTES is her first book.

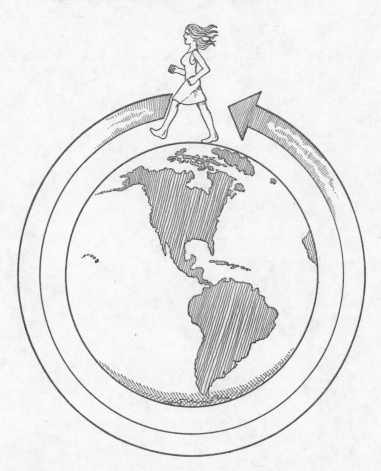